How to
Maximize
the
Caloric Costs
of
Exercise

A RELATIVELY SHORT STORY

Christopher B. Scott, PhD
Professor, Exercise Science

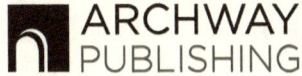
ARCHWAY
PUBLISHING

Archway Publishing books may be ordered through booksellers or by contacting:

Archway Publishing
1663 Liberty Drive
Bloomington, IN 47403
www.archwaypublishing.com
1 (888) 242-5904

ISBN: 978-1-4808-5335-5 (sc)
ISBN: 978-1-4808-5336-2 (hc)
ISBN: 978-1-4808-5334-8 (e)

Library of Congress Control Number: 2017918435

Print information available on the last page.

Archway Publishing rev. date: 12/12/2017

This book is dedicated to:

JACK LALANNE & RICHARD SIMMONS

In my time, they best personified the
importance of physical movement.

Contents

Introduction

Calorie counting, fat burning and how exercise may best achieve both are the subject matter described within these pages. From television sets to textbooks, the topic of weight loss is certainly portrayed with as much folklore as science. Nowadays, we can add the internet as a source of guidance. Wherever it is found, a majority of available information clearly advocates that diet (nutrition), not exercise, far better achieves the goal of weight loss – and I agree. So why place a focus on exercise? Because exercise helps. And you should never forget about the benefits to health and well-being that regular physical activity also provides, they are nothing short of remarkable.

Truthfully, while an ardent exercise-follower, I was not much of a fan of aerobic dance, I was more of the stereotypical weight lifting and running guy – the Jack LaLanne type. This text also is dedicated to Richard Simmons because I knew full well, at a relatively early age, just what he represented and how importantly he was needed in a society that was growing ever-increasingly sedentary. During my first two years in college, I majored in physical education, not too far from the exercise physiologist I am today. Young and naïve at the time, I still clearly recall an Introduction to Physical Education lecture where one of the first things scrawled on the chalkboard was the statement:

Failure = Quit

I've put quite a bit of thought into that proclamation over the years and so too, I'm sure, did Jack LaLanne and Richard Simmons. They understood the significance of regular physical movement and more importantly, brought that message to the masses, not just the beautiful and buff amongst us. How significantly? Profoundly so. Fit, fat or performance-impaired, one's physical activity must of necessity be something you choose to do because it is most profoundly linked to both physical and psychological well-being.

Regular physical activity creates a myriad of physiological changes within the human body, almost all of it good. Exercise is the heart and soul of physical and athletic development. The book you are reading however is not about that; you'll need to read about the enhancement of muscular performance elsewhere. This is a book about the hows and whys of counting calories with the ultimate achievement of losing body fat. I am in fact, at a current understanding that exercise designed to increase athletic ability does not necessarily carry-over to weight loss – the goals of weight reduction and the enhancement of physical performance require separate program designs... but I'm getting ahead of myself.

As part of my learning (data collection) and teaching (data promoting) background, I count calories for a living and have been happily at it for over 30 years. The following chapters present energy cost estimates – aka, calories (kcal) burned - based on numbers collected from actual laboratory measurements as well as speculative interpretations that have all been converted into an energy cost and fat loss appraisal: More vs. Less.

I continue to search for those specific types of exercises and activities that yield the largest calories-burned numbers. My primary objective is to find those physical movements with the potential to maximize caloric costs and all with the ultimate goal of losing body fat.

It is not a straightforward story...

I.

Where You Are...

Exercise scientists like me continue to pursue gold standards. One such example is the determination of the *minimum* amount of exercise or activity required to promote a healthy well-being. From a 'how much' perspective, a figure of about 1000 calories per week has perhaps been most prominently cited; burn about 150 calories (kcal) per day in physical activity and your health benefits from exercise are covered. Yet from the standpoint of weight loss, how many calories a person *chooses* to willingly expend as well as the selection of a specific exercise routine is a bit more subjective. In terms of exercise structure or design, an effort can indeed be made to create programs that attempt to *maximize* caloric cost and fat loss. And within these pages you won't need a calculator to do so. Based on the application of concepts, I attempt to describe how and why the manipulation of physical movement effects the associated energy cost; how in relative terms to maximize calories burned. In truth however, both bias and science are at play here and each requires justification.

Whether a high school dropout or a PhD scientist, much if not all of what you think you know about exercise (or just about anything else for that matter) comes from a principal source, usually the first thing you were told. Lather. Rinse. Repeat. The next generation off that grapevine follows suit, often repeating verbatim the same guidelines they themselves were taught. Or perhaps with a few added variations and terminology twists that deliver a new and/or improved appearance. In academia for example, a very specific type of physical movement known as steady state exercise – walking, jogging, bicycling and the like – has been studied rather intensely within exercise science laboratories around the globe. Many of us understand this type of exercise design with the adjective 'aerobics'. The subsequent result of decades of investigation into aerobic exercise provides the current standard regarding the how's and why's of exercise induced caloric expenditure and fat loss. It is without question a worldwide standard.

Want to know how many calories it takes to walk or jog a mile? That's already been figured out for you. While body weight, walking speeds, as well as hills and valleys certainly affect the outcome, an estimate can be provided of about 4.0 to 4.5 kcal per minute. Want to lose a pound of fat?

1 gram of fat = ~9.0 kcal
1 pound of fat = ~4000 kcal

At 4000 kcal per pound and 4 calories per minute of exercise, it would take a walk or series of walks over a 16-plus hour period to lose that pound. This knowledge and more was derived from the rather comprehensive studies of aerobic steady state exercise, also referred to as aerobic endurance or cardiovascular training. And it's all good stuff to be sure, because it works. Academic organizations like the American College of Sports Medicine (ACSM) claim tens of thousands of members world-wide and the fitness industry with its multitude of organized and globalized peoples, likely numbers in the hundreds of millions, all preaching the known virtues of aerobic exercise.

When I was in school, we were told that in order for exercise to be beneficial in the energy cost, fat burning and health-related departments, you pretty much had to become a distance runner, or at the very least some kind of an endurance athlete. Cardiovascular exercise requires the use of large muscle masses (typically those muscles from the waist down), moving at a low to moderate intensity, in a continuous and rhythmic pattern over an extended period of time – running and bicycling! Cardiovascular exercise consumes large volumes of oxygen and indeed, the maximum rate of oxygen a person consumes during all-out treadmill or cycling exercise has been used as the greatest of fitness & health scores – the beloved VO_2 max measurement. The higher your VO_2 max score, the better your health and fitness levels were presumed to be.

In many ways aerobic steady state exercise still rules the scientific realms of fitness and health because that's where it all started and in a large part remains.

But what about the caloric costs and fat loss properties of those exercises and activities that are not steady state in nature? Take for example the current and very popular interest in higher intensity intermittent exercise, activities that typically involve strength, speed and/or high power output lasting for seconds, not minutes or hours. Moreover, some sort of recovery period follows each intermittent exercise bout that subsequently allows you to resume another high intensity bout or set. In fact, intermittent exercise has as many recovery periods as it does exercise. Although you can say the same for a single bout of steady state exercise, having only one recovery period, there are unquestionable differences between the two that require both recognition and subsequent interpretation.

Resistance or weight training may best represent intermittent exercise. A typical weight lifting set may last 30 seconds or so, with a recovery period between sets lasting a few to several minutes. Three sets, three recovery periods, five sets, five recovery periods, ten sets, ten recovery periods – under steady state conditions one exercise period is followed by one recovery period. I am under the impression that steady state exercise and intermittent non-steady exercises are also different in the caloric cost and fat burning departments – very different.

As I've learned and practiced over the years, it is apparent that so-called measurements of energy costs are not what they seem. When you see a measure of caloric costs anywhere, in published form or perhaps on the electronic console of a treadmill or cycle ergometer or the app you wear, that number must be recognized as an indirect estimate at best, it is most certainly not a direct measurement. Understanding that there are more ways to skin this 'energy cost cat', I began to examine higher intensity intermittent exercises from a standpoint different from that of lower intensity steady state exercise. At this early stage of the game it's been a risk to be sure and one that has not been well received by those who continue to adhere to what I'll call traditional steady state science.

It now appears, and there's a lot of accumulating anecdotal evidence and published research to suggest, that just a few minutes of higher intensity intermittent exercise per day, a few to several times per week, can cause rather drastic and favorable changes to human physiology and health. More so than low-to-moderate steady state aerobic exercise, this looks promising because higher intensity intermittent exercise may burn more fat calories as compared to its lower intensity steady state counterpart. Within these pages I attempt to explain why.

Beyond the myopic view of the steady state regimen there are certainly other forms of human movement that need a total makeover approach to investigation. I have taken a perspective of caloric expenditure that is more specific to brief bouts or sets of higher intensity intermittent exercise. We did not apply what was learned through the study of lower intensity, steady state, continuous exercise, toward the estimation of the caloric costs of higher intensity, non-steady state, intermittent exercise. Our model has drawn accolades from some and opposition from others. And that's OK. That's how science actually works.

Rudyard Kipling wrote about the imposters that both triumph and disaster were (the poem, "If-") – they aptly describe my trials and tribulations. Indeed, my energy cost interpretations have resulted in requested presentations at several International venues, all expenses paid (Triumph!). In fact, the director of one overseas conference told me I was there because in contrast to everything else he was reading regarding the caloric costs of high intensity intermittent exercise, I'd done things correctly. On the other hand, I had an editor of a most influential exercise science journal call to inform me that they would not consider publishing anything regarding my energy cost model (Disaster!), banning it from the scientific review process altogether (during this "courtesy call" I was politely told to save my application fee). This is without question science at work.

The chapters that follow each contain boldfaced take home messages and for this chapter that message is:

The information presented within this text describes how the modification of physical movement can help maximize caloric costs and fat burning.

II.

Move!

Muscles contract, they work by becoming shorter, that's what they're best known for. Yet muscles do so much more, they further act as springs, struts, shock absorbers and brakes. In fact, muscles are recruited to perform a wonderfully diverse set of tasks. One of the first persons to not only understand this but *apply* it to exercise design was none other than Charles Atlas.

As a kid I distinctly recall on the back inside cover of many a comic book, the story of a scrawny 97-pound weakling who gets sand kicked in his face by the local beach bully, losing a romantic prospect in the process. The answer to such problems was of course a strength and development program that could transform scrawny losers into well-muscled heroes. Charles Atlas was credited with the design of this physical enhancement program that in addition to actually working, is still considered one of the better advertising campaigns of all time.

Born Angelo Siciliano (1892-1972) and later legally changing his name to what many now remember, Charles Atlas, so the story goes, watched lions and tigers at a zoo and wondered exactly how they developed the musculature they had. Resistance training was certainly around at that point in time but as Mr. Atlas concluded, none of these animals was a weight lifter. He did note however, that they stretched, flexed, preened and pawed, amid an endless variety of other sorts of physical prowess and performance. Charles Atlas was on to something, what he called *dynamic tension*. Dynamic tension requires an explanation of the 3 basic types of muscle recruitment because it represents combinations of three types of muscular "work": isometric, isotonic and isokinetic.

Isometric may be the easiest term to understand as it requires the contraction of muscle, but with no physical movement. Put your hands together in front of your chest and push hard – force is produced but if no movement took place, the exercise is termed isometric. Wall squats (a sitting position held in place with your back against a wall) and planks (holding the body in a push-up position) are further examples of isometric exercises. There are many, many others.

It is of interest that just as Mr. Atlas was coming into his own (1920's-1930's) the academic-types were investigating energy related questions regarding contracting skeletal muscle (frog muscle to be exact). What they found laid the groundwork for our current understanding of what is now known as the force-velocity relationship. In fact, the greatest force muscle can apply is when it is not moving – an isometric contraction.

An isotonic contraction consists of actual movement. As a muscle shortens and contracts, force is applied and weight is lifted in what is known as a concentric contraction. A muscle that is lengthening with force – the lowering of that weight – undergoes an eccentric contraction. Lower energy costs are associated with eccentric contractions; concentric contractions require a greater caloric cost. As an example, climbing stairs (concentric work) is much more expensive as compared to walking down them (eccentric work). Physical movement almost always requires both and then some - remember, brakes, springs, struts and shock absorbers are all within muscles resume.

With isokinetic work, movement speed affects contractile force: muscle applies less force the faster the movement; with slower movement speeds, an increased force can be applied. Movement speed is further addressed in subsequent chapters as it has a rather significant effect on overall costs.

Given the maximal potential for force production when not moving, isometric muscle contractions are ideal for gaining strength and that's a great thing. However, a problem that arises with isometric exercise is that there is no range of motion in an isometric contraction, so that strength gains are limited to the position the limbs are held in as they apply force. Sadly, there's another more serious pitfall. From an energy cost perspective isometric contractions are problematic in that they reveal the lowest overall caloric cost as compared to isotonic and isokinetic conditions. Why is this?

At the molecular level a protein called *myosin* is what enables muscle contraction to take place. Myosin is a well-known molecular motor of sorts that kind of looks like the business end of a golf club, with the head of the club being able to move or "ratchet" fore and aft. It's certainly well known that muscle requires energy to contract but that explanation is in fact so simplistic, it is in reality incorrect.

In its natural *lowest* energy state, myosin actually holds itself in a contracted position. Energy is required for myosin to position itself in an un-contracted state, one of *higher* energy. So, with no movement taking place – an isometric contraction - myosin is actually demanding less energy. No doubt the best example of this phenomenon occurs a few to several hours after death when the body's musculature goes into the state of *rigor mortis*, when all muscles are fully rigid, undergoing complete contracture. With death, every cell in your body loses energy exchange abilities and without energy, muscle goes into its natural state of contracture (days later, decomposition rules as the reign of *rigor mortis* ends).

Another way to look at this is understanding that muscular work is a product of physical force and displacement (movement!) and with no motion taking place, the amount of work completed is little to none and so too is the energy cost.

The take home message: regarding the 3 types of muscular work:

Maximizing energy costs comes with physical movement, <u>not</u> isometric force production

One of our investigations involved the estimation of energy costs for 3 types of intermittent exercise training routines. Each carefully controlled exercise routine lasted 4 minutes; the words *carefully controlled* means a specific time-controlled cadence was adhered to. The reference and its accompanying modified abstract is posted below in typical science journal jargon:

> "Total energy costs of 3...calisthenic squatting routines: isometric, isotonic and jump, *European Journal of Human Movement*, 35:34-40, 2015".

> We examined the total energy costs – aerobic and anaerobic, exercise and recovery – of three...squat routines: isotonic, isometric and plyometric (jump

or isokinetic). Our intent was to determine which format elicited the greatest overall cost. **Materials and Methods**: Four male and three female subjects volunteered (23.7 ± 2.6 years, 170.1 ± 10.3 cm, 68.2 ± 14.6 kg). Isotonic and jump squats were completed in 20 second bouts at a cadence of 2 seconds per squat (10 repetitions each) followed by 10 seconds of recovery; isometric squats were held for the entirety of each 20 second exercise period followed by 10 seconds of recovery – exercise and recovery bouts were repeated 8 times for a total of 4 minutes. **Results and Discussion**: Jump squats had the greatest overall energy cost at 38 kcal followed by isotonic squats at 27 kcal; there was no statistical difference between the two. Isometric squats at 15 kcal were significantly lower than both isotonic and jump squats. From an exercise program design standpoint isometric exercises do not appear to represent an appropriate format when attempting to maximize energy costs.

Want to lose a pound of fat? Just repeat the 4-minute isometric squat format provided above 267 times for about 18 hours overall and you're there! Or, as mentioned earlier, you could walk for 16-plus miles. As will be repeated throughout these pages, these choices and more are yours...

It is important to mention that another measurement was taken for the squat routines and that measure was the rating of perceived exertion (RPE). Perceived exertion reflects muscular effort and physical sensation in relation to the exercise being performed. The scale was created by Gunnar Borg, a Swedish psychologist and physiologist and his original *Borg Scale* looks like this:

6	No exertion at all
7	Extremely light
8	
9	Very light
10	
11	Light
12	
13	Somewhat hard
14	
15	Hard (heavy)
16	
17	Very hard
18	
19	Extremely hard
20	Maximal exertion

The Borg scale was originally created based on heart rate responses to what is known as steady state exercise, typically bicycling. Placing a zero after each of the numbers displayed above would provide an approximation of heart rate at that level of steady state (cardiovascular) physical exertion.

For our 3 types of well-controlled squat routines, the highest ratings of perceived exertion came with the jump and isometric squats, at a rating of 'somewhat hard'. For the isotonic squat, the perceived exertion was rated between 'very light' and 'light'. Isometric exercise routines are thought by many to be somewhat difficult, whereby the holding of muscle in a non-moving contracted state becomes uncomfortable over time and emotional descriptions that invoke pain and suffering are the result. But while that misery is accompanied by emotional duress and a higher heart rate, a greater caloric cost does not follow. As compared to an isometric muscle contraction, start moving (isotonic or isokinetic movement) and perceived exertion and heart rate can actually <u>drop</u> as energy costs accrue. The ramifications here in terms of exercise program design and the maximization of energy costs are important:

An exercise or activity that is perceived as being difficult does not necessarily correlate with increased energy costs.

It is also apparent that heart rate and energy costs are not always perfectly related. Consider a distance running champion and a sedentary couch-potato both together taking a 1-mile stroll. At an identical body weight the caloric cost would likewise be similar for both, but the heart rate of each would be quite different - perhaps 60-something for the athlete and 100-and-something for the potato. A measurement of heart rate can help or hinder an exercise energy cost estimate.

One last mention concerning perceived exertion: at an overseas strength and conditioning convention held in Madrid, Spain, Gary Hunter from the University of Alabama (Birmingham) presented information regarding a given person's weight or body fat gains over a period of time. Dr. Hunter has been at it for a while too, with five decades of data collection and analysis to his credit. After careful examination of the many data sets his team has collected, the highest correlation found with chronic weight gain over time was... perceived exertion. Wow. What a thought or perhaps more appropriately, what an attitude. If you regard exercise, activity, or physical movement in general as an unpleasant overly-strenuous exertion (for whatever reason, legitimate or not), you will likely be gaining weight in the coming years. And conceivably some or much of that can be prevented by *choosing* to be active.

Think of physical movement beyond isometric muscle contraction. If you're sitting as you read this you are of course applying sitting-muscle-forces, but you are not moving; your energy demands are minimal. If you are standing and reading, bravo; but your daily costs of living still reside in the minimization category, albeit in the upper echelons of that classification.

Think physical movement, then do it. Think in terms of regular episodes of *chosen* physical activity over the course of a day, a week, a lifetime:

Want to maximize energy costs? Move!

III.

Law of the Land: The Aerobic Steady State Energy Cost

Our ability to consume oxygen that provides energy to working muscle, in fact to all of our cells, is called aerobic metabolism. Oxygen is well recognized as an absolute requirement for survival. But oxygen is also dangerous stuff. While clearly necessary to support life, over the course of a lifetime oxygen is quite literally killing us too. Oxygen is regarded as being extremely electronegative, a molecular-bully property that invokes the snatching of electrons from other molecules. Iron degrades by rusting, its deterioration being a direct result of its contact with oxygen. We likewise age as the oxygen we breathe grabs electrons from our cells' DNA and the many other molecules that life is comprised of. That's when wrinkles, liver spots, grey hair and yellow toenails begin to make their appearances. Thanks for everything and nothing, oxygen.

Oxygen consumption *measurements* are the current gold standard in the service of *estimating* energy costs. Exercise scientists use the acronym VO_2 to signify the volume (V) of oxygen (O_2) consumed, typically in a liters per minute format ($1 \cdot min^{-1}$). In the late 1960s a medical doctor by the name of Ken Cooper coined the term *aerobics* to describe exercise and activities that require large volumes of oxygen. The word stuck and it is now difficult to go anywhere in the world where the word aerobics is not understood.

Aerobic is the standard descriptor of cardiovascular-oriented oxygen consuming exercise. Moreover, for the practicing exercise scientist, aerobic exercise represents the very foundation of how the link between fitness and health was forged. Indeed, a person's VO_2 max – a representation of one's maximum ability to take in and utilize oxygen during all-out aerobic exercise – was once considered the be all and end all marker of a person's health and fitness. The higher your VO_2 max, the more fit you were considered and the healthier you were supposed to be. We now know that well-being and physical prowess are a bit more complicated. As an example, while VO_2 max is indeed a useful identification of the capacity of your lungs and heart to take in and deliver oxygen, it does not represent peak muscular work or power output.

Here's another interpretation: Usain Bolt has run 100 meters in 9.58 seconds (23.26 mph), which as an aerobic feat would require an implausibly large, physiologically impossible VO_2 max, and yet the fastest human being on planet Earth is not a successful endurance athlete. He can however operate at an exercise *intensity* that is well over *twice* that of your standard gym-rat VO_2 max. Make no mistake, peak skeletal muscle power and force output resides well above cardiovascular oxygen-delivery capabilities; in this realm, energy undergoes exchange via anaerobic mechanisms. We'll get to anaerobic metabolism in later chapters, but for the moment let's get back to low to moderate intensity aerobic territory.

Caloric costs are typically presented as a per minute estimate taken directly from a per minute oxygen consumption measurement, setting the stage for pretty much all energy cost descriptions of exercise in terms of 60 second time periods. That is, an estimate of calories per minute is converted from a measurement of oxygen consumed per minute. Aerobic exercise is considered steady state when the intensity, work rate or power output do not fluctuate over time. Minute-by-minute, the oxygen consumed and the calories expended are considered proportionate – a steady state.

It's actually not at all difficult to measure oxygen consumption. Oxygen and carbon dioxide exchanges are collected with a mouthpiece or mask placed over the mouth, with subsequent analysis by a device that measures respiratory gas exchange known as a *metabolic cart*. As connected to a personal computer, the metabolic cart provides almost instantaneous descriptions of oxygen uptake and carbon dioxide and it all takes place with the push of a button. In fact, an energy expenditure treatise written decades ago stated specifically that the largest errors in the course of caloric cost estimation come from a failure to correctly determine the length of time spent in any activity and not the oxygen-related assessment of the cost of that activity. This is likely true for low to moderate intensity aerobic exercises that primarily rely on oxygen, but not so for intermittent strength, speed and high power output that may not. Indeed, the unintended and improper usage of steady state measurements as applied to non-steady state, intermittent exercise serves as the primary impetus for writing this text. So why is the aerobic, oxygen consuming, steady state so authoritative to exercise scientists?

Aerobic energy cost estimates are derived from steady state cardiovascular exercise, where large muscle masses undergo continuous, rhythmic, steady rate contractions for a relatively lengthy period of time, typically 20 to 60 minutes. Walking, jogging, and cycling - the quintessential aerobic exercises - are easily studied with treadmills and bicycle ergometers; the standard equipment that resides within most exercise science and human performance laboratories. Unfortunately, while the type of effort – speed and grade – are easily identified with the treadmill, exactly how much work is being performed is difficult to quantify.

Put simply, physics defines work as [force x vertical displacement] so that if you are running on a level surface, little to no work is completed, but clearly you're doing something in terms of caloric cost. On the contrary, bicycle ergometers are quite good at measuring power output (Watts), a rather exacting measurement. Regardless, both tools set the precedent for the energy cost assessment of *all* formats of exercise, steady state or not.

If a bicyclists' power output were to remain constant and a measure of oxygen uptake for that work rate was also found to be constant, then the steady state oxygen uptake can be considered a valid match to the steady rate of power. Steady state oxygen uptake measurements of steady rate aerobic exercise are correctly considered valid – the so-called *gold standard* of energy cost estimations. And scientists cannot work without valid measurements.

The next figure reveals the steady state consumption of oxygen (in a per liter format: liters $O_2 \cdot min^{-1}$) for a person walking on a treadmill at four different steady rate speeds: **1)** 2.0, **2)** 2.5, **3)** 3.0 and **4)** 3.5 miles per hour.

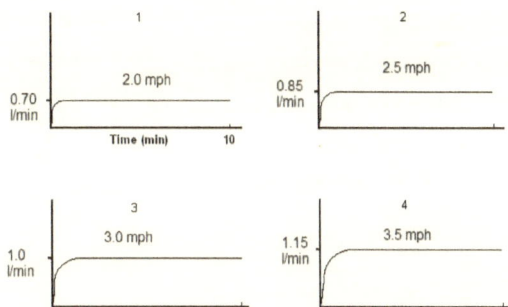

The measurement of oxygen uptake in a steady state, liters per minute format is shown above for 4 separate steady state treadmill walks at 4 different speeds. Note that at the start of exercise a few minutes are required until a steady rate of oxygen uptake is achieved. The steady state is portrayed as a non-changing, flat horizontal line.

Once the oxygen uptake for any walking speed is collected, another graph can be drawn revealing the oxygen uptake relationship for each walking speed. The data clearly reveals that the greater the walking speed or intensity, the proportionately greater rate at which oxygen is consumed. As the next figure indicates, a straight-forward linear relationship is revealed.

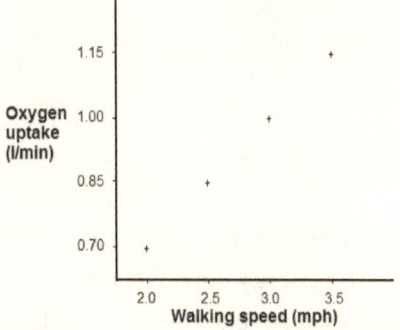

The 4 oxygen uptake data points taken from 4 walking speeds can be portrayed as a straight line, demonstrating a predictable linear relationship between oxygen consumed per minute for any and all walking speeds.

Estimations or predictions are made easier with straight lines. In fact, once a few data points are collected at slow to moderate walking speeds, an extrapolation can be made for any speed of forward locomotion; walking, jogging, running or sprinting. See the next figure...

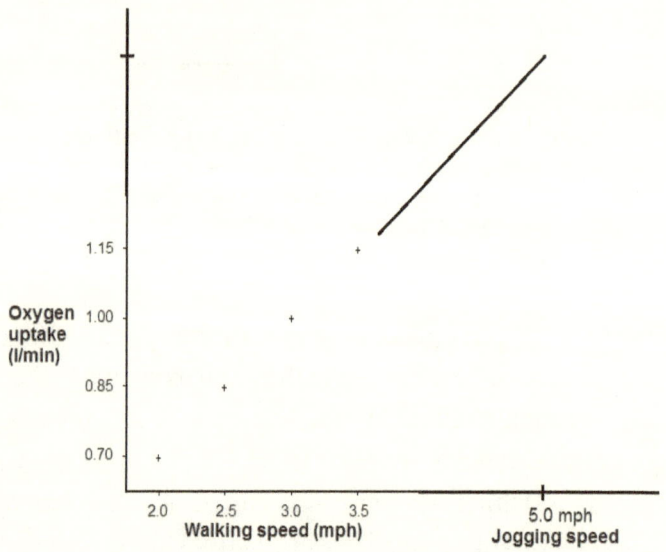

Because of the linearity seen between steady state lower intensity aerobic exercise and oxygen uptake, the energy costs associated with faster speeds can be estimated quite easily by simply extrapolating a straight line from the four data points. Increase aerobic exercise intensity and energy costs are assumed to follow suit in a very predictable fashion, from walking to jogging, running to sprinting.

Note carefully however what the steady state *exercise* model does not portray: the energy cost of the *recovery* from exercise. Any measurement of recovery oxygen uptake is typically kept separate from that of steady state exercise and for good reason. Recovery oxygen uptake is not in a steady state, falling exponentially toward resting levels the moment aerobic exercise stops.

Average the steady state oxygen uptake of exercise with the plummeting non-steady oxygen consumed in recovery, and the overall per minute estimated cost is actually lowered. Recovery costs need to be added to the exercise costs, not averaged.

Oxygen uptake is shown above for an extended period of aerobic steady state exercise followed by recovery. Note that for the first few minutes at the start of exercise, oxygen uptake rises until a steady state rate of oxygen consumption is achieved. Following exercise, a single recovery period is shown where non-steady state oxygen uptake falls exponentially towards resting levels (at low to moderate exercise intensities it is debatable whether or not recovery contributes significantly to overall energy costs).

Minus the energy costs of recovery, published exercise energy cost estimates must be understood as being somewhat incomplete. But clearly, knowledge of the exercise cost alone is a great start and most certainly useful.

There is a further reality to the energy cost-steady state exercise relationship that requires clarification. Careful and repeated measurements of oxygen uptake for a given individual at any specific gait – walking, jogging, running and sprinting - actually reveal that per minute energy costs are not linear across all speeds, they are in fact slightly curvilinear. This is, in my opinion, more of a limitation than a problem. The next figure dramatizes the opposite ends of the so-called caloric cost-to-intensity straight line that actually has slight curvature at the slowest and faster speeds.

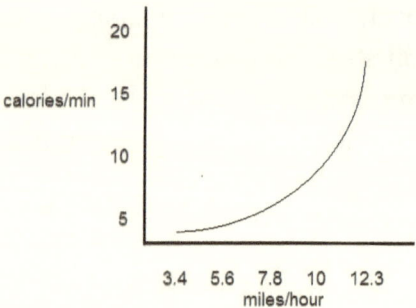

In the figure above, the energy costs of 2-legged locomotion develop a non-linearity at slower and faster speeds. Even so, most all published estimates of the caloric cost of exercise assume a linear relationship between intensity and energy costs and that's not a bad thing at all.

In terms of energy cost interpretation, the difference between an indirect estimate and a direct measurement must be recognized: oxygen uptake serves as the direct measurement, the caloric-cost-to-exercise-intensity-straight-line-interpretation serves as the accepted estimate (minus the recovery cost).

The American College of Sports Medicine (ACSM) has published perhaps the most definitive guidelines in regard to the energy costs of walking and running. Being authorities on the subject, they state that linear models utilizing per minute units are the preferred methodology of choice – indeed, what is considered the only valid measure - for estimating the costs of forward locomotion specific to walking and moderate running speeds. Yet take a closer look at the next figure… in a comparison of walking and running, absolute linearity between speed and cost is a bit of an illusion.

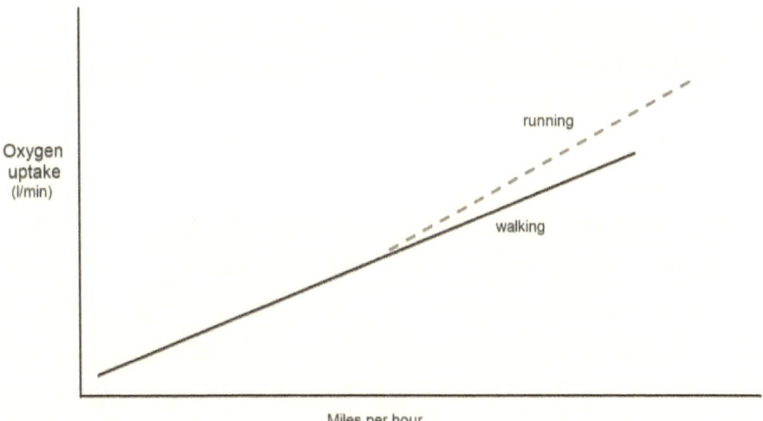

*As demonstrated above, per minute oxygen uptake
measurements are maximized with running as opposed
to walking. It does not take a stretch of the imagination to
recognize that the two straight lines shown above collectively
reveal a single slightly curved line: as speed (intensity)
increases, costs can actually rise disproportionately.*

The linear format of a steady state energy cost estimate is
inherent to old and new technologies alike. Take 'wearables' for
instance, those devices that can be applied to cell phones, body-
wear, bracelets and sneakers, which collect data and provide an
estimate of exercise energy costs. It all typically begins within
an Exercise Science Laboratory of some kind where a group of
subjects, performing a specific exercise, undergoes an oxygen
uptake measurement. The business side of the fitness industry,
utilizing the latest in Information Technology research and
development, creates the tools – heart rate monitors, motion
detectors, accelerometers (3D motion detectors), heat sensors,
pedometers and phone apps – that were originally connected
directly or indirectly to a per minute oxygen uptake measurement. These devices offer reasonable to erroneous energy cost
estimates for low to moderate intensity steady state aerobic

exercise, perhaps most incorrectly for higher intensity intermittent exercise.

But that's a good start.

Right or wrong, all this energy cost technology initiates an interest into tracking daily physical activity and more, and that's a very, very, very good thing. Have you moved(!) today?

Error and variability: this is the very nature of the energy cost guestimation business. And there is nothing bad about that. Scientists call this predicament not right or wrong but instead a limitation from where we can still draw informative conclusions. Here's one that everybody can agree on:

From a cost per minute aerobic perspective, increases in exercise intensity maximize caloric costs.

There are however, other approaches to the examination of energy costs; exercise need not be viewed solely from per minute steady state perspectives. The next chapter begins the description of why.

IV.

No-Man's Land: The Anaerobic Threshold

Exercising at a specific steady state power output or work rate, a specific amount of muscle is recruited to perform at that specific intensity. At a low to moderate intensity, exercise can last for hours but as you are likely well aware, higher intensities will eventually promote fatigue, typically in seconds or minutes, steady state or not. In fact, a line of demarcation has been drawn that separates higher exercise intensity from its lower to moderate exertion counterparts: that boundary is known as the anaerobic threshold. To better approach the energy costs of higher intensity activity beyond the anaerobic threshold, it is important to understand the basic qualities or types of skeletal muscle.

Physiologists have described 3 categories of skeletal muscle: fast twitch, slow twitch and somewhere in-between twitches, where the characteristics of a muscle fibers' contraction speed are being identified. As any physical movement is initiated, your nervous system at first recruits smaller slower twitch fibers and these muscle fibers are primarily aerobic in nature, they excel at the consumption of oxygen (oxidizing glucose and fat as fuel). As exercise intensity increases or if you rapidly dive-into an extreme bout of exercise, both slow twitch and larger faster twitch muscle fibers are recruited to perform the task at hand.

Strength! Speed! Power! These events are owned and operated by fast twitch muscle fibers. The energy exchange metabolism of fast twitch muscle is considered mostly anaerobic, less so aerobic, and a preferred fuel is the limited storage of the glucose found within. Glucose is stored in most all cells as glycogen, the 3-dimensional structure actually resembles a kooshball of stringed-together molecules. Needing fuel fast, muscles engaged in higher intensity exercise briskly consume their glycogen (glucose) stores, foregoing oxygen consumption and instead producing lactic acid as energy is rapidly and anaerobically harvested - the splitting of a single glucose molecule into two molecules of lactic acid is called *glycolysis*.

1 molecule of glucose ($C_6H_{12}O_6$) =
2 molecules of lactic acid ($C_3H_6O_3$)

The provision of energy as our muscle cells "burn" glucose and fat is certainly a marvelous thing, but aerobic metabolism is somewhat limited in terms of the speed of energy provision (again, VO_2 max is <u>not</u> an energy cost max). Glucose and glycogen can be broken down without any need for oxygen and that anaerobic metabolic process is exceedingly fast, much faster than aerobic metabolism. For all who enjoy those sports and activities that are associated with strength, speed and high power output, that's great news. Yet all-out strength and speed comes with a price and the initiation of those extra expenses originates with and after the anaerobic threshold.

The progression of exercise intensity may be best explained with a treadmill test to exhaustion. In the determination of heart health, your doctor may hook you up to an electrocardiogram (ECG) and ask you to walk or jog on a treadmill, where every few minutes the speed and/or grade are increased. The treadmill always wins too. For a test to exhaustion that's where the fun ends, quite literally when you can't take another step. As you continue along the light exercise to maximal exertion spectrum more muscle is recruited to complete the burgeoning challenge at hand, and as you begin to recruit large faster twitch muscles you initiate a trip down that road called 'Fatigue'.

Actual measurement of the anaerobic threshold requires an assessment of blood lactic acid levels or the measurement of oxygen and carbon dioxide exchanges using a metabolic cart. For those lacking these abilities, at some point along the rising exercise intensity continuum you will start to feel a bit winded, typically at a perceived exertion of 'somewhat hard to hard' and can no longer talk with ease; the anaerobic threshold resides in this territory.

For most active adults, the anaerobic threshold is found at an intensity of about 55-60% of a VO_2 max measurement (where, of course, 100% VO_2 max is considered the maximal rate of *aerobic* energy exchange). That means that someone in decent physical condition can perform steady state exercise at or below an intensity of about 50% of VO_2 max for perhaps several hours. World class endurance athletes – marathon runners are a perfect example – can race at about a 2-hour, 26-mile pace at 85-90% of VO_2 max, an amazingly impressive feat (but make no mistake, up the intensity ante to 91% of VO_2 max and that race ends differently).

The anaerobic threshold was originally defined as that specific exercise intensity where the oxygen supply or delivery to working muscle became compromised - muscle was thought to become anaerobic at that very point. Professor George Brooks at the University of California at Berkeley changed all that with a focus not on the supply of oxygen, but instead with the increased recruitment of larger, more powerful, less-efficient, faster twitch muscle fibers. When called on for active duty, fast twitch muscle fuels itself by rapidly and anaerobically splitting glucose molecules into two molecules of lactic acid. And as mentioned earlier, it all takes place several hundred-fold faster than the provision of energy supplied by aerobic oxygen consuming metabolism.

To be sure, fast twitch muscle can and does consume oxygen, but its motor is best run via an anaerobic, lactic acid-producing metabolism. In fact, the anaerobic threshold is always identified as part of an oxygen uptake measurement at a percentage of VO_2 max. Even so, the growing appearance of accumulating lactic acid not only helps further demonstrate the concept of the so-called anaerobic threshold, it also suggests the accumulation of anaerobic energy costs in addition to those associated with oxygen uptake.

From an energy cost perspective, higher intensity exercise most certainly burns more calories, yet the anaerobic threshold is where the linear guestimation of energy exchange begins to breakdown. To be sure, at low to moderate intensity steady state exercise, our energy cost estimates are pretty good. But above the anaerobic threshold the estimation of energy costs is a crap shoot because that threshold is a self-serving measurement. It can be different for everyone as are the rising contributions of non-steady state energy costs – aerobic and anaerobic.

Active fitness enthusiast or world champion athlete, a person's energy costs begin to rise as the anaerobic threshold is breached, even as the power output or work rate stays the same (a steady state). At work rates and power outputs beyond the anaerobic threshold, further curves are added to the supposed linear work-to-energy cost relationship (see the next figure). This is the very fly in the energy cost ointment; at any given level of higher intensity steady state exercise, the energy cost is not the same for all, measures and estimates be damned.

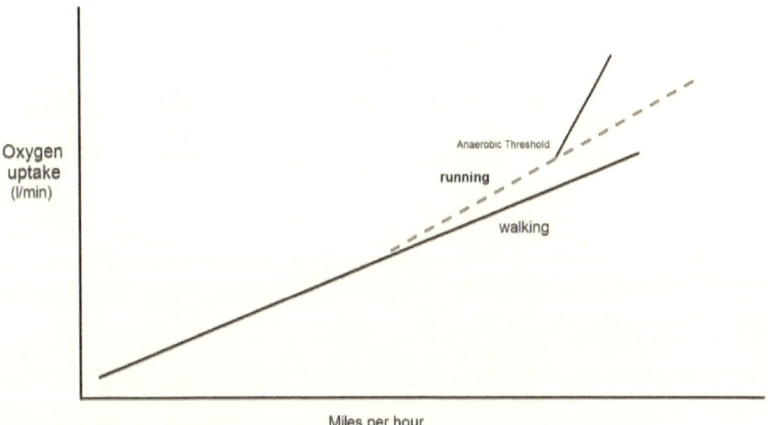

The anaerobic threshold is shown above for running. At that running speed at which the threshold occurs, aerobic and anaerobic energy costs begin to rise in a non-linear disproportional format which differs among people, the result of the recruitment of more and inefficient larger fast twitch muscle fibers. As muscular recruitment progresses, so too do the associated energy costs, adding yet another curve(s) to the supposed steady state energy cost straight line.

The anaerobic threshold and beyond is an energy cost no-man's land:

At and above the anaerobic threshold, energy costs cannot be determined with validity – higher intensity exercise helps maximize caloric costs, but how much so is questionable at best.

Time to start thinking outside the box.

V.

A Different Perspective: Energy Costs Per Task

Sometimes you just have to look at something differ-ently to obtain a more complete understanding. Take for instance the expression of exercise and liters of oxygen consumed not in terms of per minute measurements, but instead as the amount of oxygen necessary to complete a specific physical task, steady state or not.

As an example, walking, jogging or running 1 mile can be viewed in the context of a single task - as the energy cost per mile (not cost per minute). As a generalized rule of thumb, forward locomotion requires approximately 100 kcal per mile. If true, the task of walking or running a marathon (26.2 miles) has an energy cost estimated at 2,620 kcal (slightly more than the energy contained within a half-pound of fat). Steady state analyses suggest that walking requires a caloric cost of about 0.77 kcal per kilogram of body weight per mile or, approx-imately 1.53 kcal per kilogram of body weight per mile for running:

Walking - 0.77 kcal kg^{-1} mile^{-1} (0.34 kcal pound^{-1} mile^{-1})
Running - 1.53 kcal kg^{-1} mile^{-1} (0.69 kcal pound^{-1} mile^{-1})

Based on the above, a 190 pound individual would actually "burn" about 65 kcal per mile walked and about 131 kcal per mile run. The average of a walking and running speed could be called "jogging" where our 190 pound man may "burn" about 100 kcal per mile. Keep in mind these values represent a gross estimate for any given person at any given speed, they're also based on per minute steady state oxygen uptake measurements.

With the dismissal of per minute portrayals, supposed linear relationships disappear altogether between the work or exercise task and its associated energy costs. In its place a U-shaped pattern emerges. Such configuration arises from equivalent tasks performed at slow, moderate, and fast speeds. For a given, specific, physical task, slower and faster speeds promote a greater caloric cost as compared to moderate speeds.

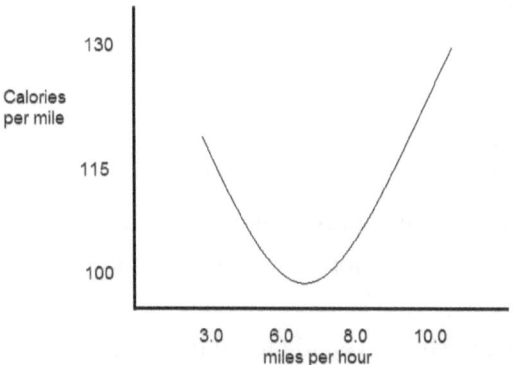

Speed has the additional effects of time and intensity on the energy costs of movement when viewed from a cost per task perspective. Over the course of 1 mile for example, walking (at 3.0 mph) and running (at 10 mph) have the highest energy costs. Jogging for 1 mile at a moderate speed (6.5 mph) actually has the lowest energy cost as compared to walking and running.

As a youngster, one of my favorite television programs was,

The Six Million Dollar Man. "We can re-build him", we were told at each shows intro, "we have the technology." The story centered on a test pilot/astronaut/secret agent by the name of Steve Austin. After surviving a horrific crash, Steve came into the possession of 2 bionic legs, a bionic right arm and a bionic left eye, and with these super-human prosthetics he performed physical miracles.

The best part of each episode however wasn't with the use of his bionic devices, but in how Agent Austin's' superhuman abilities were portrayed. Each and every time he ran 60+ miles an hour, or jumped 30 feet high, or lifted hundreds of pounds or squinted and viewed for miles and miles, the film format switched to slow motion, with terrific science-fiction sound effects to boot. And my brothers and I ate it up. Afterwards was bed time and off we *slowly* went.

Now the trip from the living room sofa to my bedroom was not all that far, even considering a flight of stairs. Most bed time excursions consisted of, perhaps, a 30 to 45 second start-to-finish, television to bed, travel-time. It wasn't too fast or too slow but a Goldilocks-like in-between speed. However, after watching *The Six Million Dollar Man*, that bedtime trip took several prolonged minutes, as we completed the whole event in the slowest of slow motion. I imagine at a moderate regular bed-time speed the task of traveling couch-to-bed was a half-calorie or so. But performing the identical task at a slower bionic-man speed, getting to bed lasted minutes not seconds, and the extra time and steps (Movement!) it took burned several calories – same task, greater cost.

The explanations for the unique U-shaped energy cost pattern – increased slower and faster costs vs. that of moderate speeds - are as follows: 1) slower speeds require more time and many more steps and therefore energy to cover a specific distance or perform a given bout or work task, and 2) faster movement speeds invoke a greater physiological intensity further increasing overall costs. In fact, your ability to walk is an unconscious reflex whose neurons reside within your spinal column; energy costs almost certainly play a role in how that reflex operates.

For any given person, a leisurely stroll invokes a natural speed, a natural stride length and a natural gait that appear to be "chosen" because of their natural amalgamation toward an upmost efficiency and the lowest cost. Change your inherently chosen walking speed, stride length or pattern of gait, and energy costs go up.

With increased speeds, a further physical component termed 'inertia' needs consideration, and with an increase in inertia comes an increase in energy demands. Earth's gravity is actually pulling you downward at an accelerated rate. When you jump and momentarily leave the surface of the earth, you have to overcome gravity's acceleration and that requires additional energy in the form of inertia (an object at rest tends to stay at rest and an object in motion tends to stay in motion until acted upon by an outside force – Sir Isaac Newton). When you land, your muscles must act as a braking system in the process of deceleration, also invoking an inertial component.

Recall the callisthenic squat routines reported earlier: squatting in preparation of jumping upwards, jumping, leaving the ground momentarily, then landing, resulted in a 30% greater caloric cost as opposed to squatting then standing upright with both feet planted firmly on the floor – this is known as a plyometric-type exercise. If the bionic man's exploits were captured in fast motion filming as opposed to slow, my parents would have likely been pleased that we achieved bed time within mere seconds as opposed to minutes. But after the physiological efforts associated with a greater speed (intensity) and the inertia related costs of plyometric-type up-and-down bounding across the floor and leaping up the stairs, it's unlikely we would have fallen asleep anytime soon.

Using cost per task analyses, a myriad of non-steady state exercises and activities can undergo examination. Per task analyses solve a noteworthy problem when investigating the costs of higher intensity exercise, where the speed and power involved cannot be maintained for lengthy periods of time. We measured, for example, the energy costs of punching a heavy bag hard-and-fast over the course of one minute. The next table compares those results with other published studies where measurements of oxygen uptake were completed over a period of several minutes to obtain a single averaged steady state per minute value. When asked to punch a heavy bag all-out for one minute, you can attack the bag with a ferocity that is much greater as compared to punching over a continuous 5 to 10-minute period where only a lower more moderate intensity can be maintained.

	For 1 minute	Average per minute
Heavy Bag Punching	30 kcal	8 – 16 kcal·min^{-1}

Punching a heavy bag all-out (highest intensity) over the time period of a single minute – 96 punches in all – resulted in an exercise and recovery oxygen uptake cost of 30 kcal. Using steady state, exercise-only methodology (excluding anaerobic and recovery costs), published estimates of heavy bag hitting reveal a lower caloric cost – you simply cannot maintain the intensity of punching for 60 seconds over an elongated 5 minute or more time period. Include the anaerobic energy costs to the 1-minute per task model and costs increase to 37 total kcal. The difference between a per task energy cost estimate and a per minute averaged exercise-only cost appears obvious.

Resistance exercise or weight training where the periods of actual activity may last seconds not minutes is yet another example of non-steady state, intermittent, high intensity exercise. Under such circumstances, the completion of a single or multiple sets of repetitions in a cost per task format may be more appropriately applied.

Moreover, a cost per task analysis can include that recovery component missing from the steady state modeling of energy costs - exercise and recovery energy cost components being added together. Another consideration is that an estimate of anaerobic energy costs is further included in the total energy cost estimation: total or overall costs are based on exercise oxygen uptake as well as recovery oxygen uptake and blood lactic acid levels. This total energy cost per task model was compared with averaged Watts to kcal per minute conversions for a one-minute bout of intense cycling:

	For 1-minute	Average per minute
250 Watts	28 kcal	$3.6 - 17.3$ kcal·min^{-1}

A search into the energy costs of bicycling reveals quite a number of published power output (Watts) to kcal per minute conversions; these values are based solely on measured oxygen uptake in minute long intervals: 3.6 – 17.3 kcal per minute. Yet begin and end a 250 Watt cycling task for 1-minute overall, and a total energy cost of 28 kcal is revealed: exercise and recovery oxygen uptake + anaerobic energy costs. Again, a per task total energy cost estimate reveals a rather substantial increase as compared to published per minute oxygen-only conversions (e.g., 1 Watt = 0.0143 kcal·min^{-1}).

Both energy cost per minute and per task models make reasonable estimates of the energy demands for many types of exercise and activity. So, for exercise and activity of all shapes and sizes, pick your poison - calories per minute or calories per task - each distorts or clarifies the truth to some extent depending on your perspective. And truth be told, neither the cost per minute nor cost per task method has achieved scientific validation in the estimation of the energy costs of brief and intense, non-steady state, intermittent exercise. Even so, many exercise scientists continue to adhere to steady state interpretations of non-steady state intermittent costs because that's what they were first taught and choose to adhere to.

Got that?

Opinions differ and it will apparently take a bit more time to reach consensus on what type of energy cost model best represents the specific conditions of higher intensity intermittent exercise and recovery. Even so:

Take any specific physical task or work bout and either slow it down or speed it up and you have just maximized the overall energy cost.

Add-in the recovery energy cost component to the overall interpretation, and we can also begin to better consider body fat and the hopeful disappearance thereof.

VI.

Stop and Go: Intermittent Exercise

Physical movement increases the amount of oxygen consumed, well above resting levels. Afterwards, upon the completion of exercise, oxygen consumption plummets rapidly back toward resting levels yet can remain elevated for a period of time. Recovery, like exercise, costs.

The recovery component of aerobic exercise has been given several names that have included: oxygen debt (an historical term), excess post-exercise oxygen consumption (EPOC) (a contemporary scientific term) and the afterburn (a mainstream fitness description).

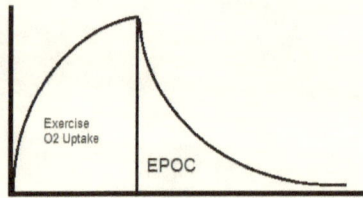

Oxygen uptake is shown during and after a single brief bout of aerobic-type exercise; this is not steady state oxygen uptake. Note that after rising quickly with exercise, recovery oxygen uptake drops precipitously downward at the end of the exercise period, yet it takes time to do so. This model is exclusive to the exercise science community, portrayed in every published exercise science textbook.

The extent of the oxygen debt/ EPOC/ afterburn has and continues to undergo extensive investigation as it is well recognized that both exercise intensity and duration drive the caloric costs of recovery, and in that order too. Aerobic exercise intensity plays a much larger role in dictating recovery costs than does exercise duration: intensity is the primary driver of recovery's energy needs.

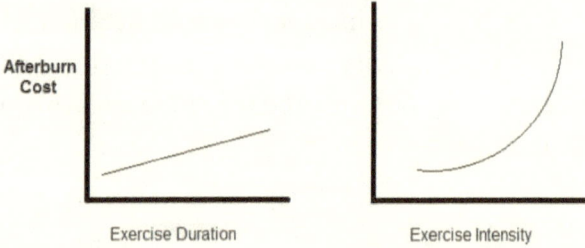

Exercise duration (at left) invokes a linear-type increase of recovery or afterburn costs; the longer the exercise period, the proportionately greater the recovery. Exercise intensity (at right) is however far-and-away the principal influence; recovery costs increase exponentially with exercise intensity (the afterburn should not be confused with an elevated day's long resting metabolic rate, which regular exercise may or more likely may not drastically improve/increase – the subject matter is very much debatable).

An elevated oxygen uptake after exercise can last minutes, hours or (wishful thinking?) perhaps days, yet regardless of the time period, the added cost is certainly contributing to the maximization of energy expenditure. And an *added* cost it is. Recall, in terms of energy cost interpretation, averaging the exercise oxygen-related cost with the recovery cost lowers the overall cost. The importance of recovery necessitates independent consideration, separate from that of exercise in order to better recognize the hows and whys of an increased ability to burn fat. A rationale for this interpretation stems from the knowledge of what fuels working and recovering skeletal muscle:

The higher the intensity of muscle contraction the more muscle relies on glucose (sugar) as a fuel - the lower the intensity, the greater the utilization of fat as a fuel.

It is now widely believed that fat may be a favored fuel during the recovery from exercise, at a time when little to no muscle contraction is taking place. It then follows that the afterburn period represents a window of opportunity for reducing body fat – more recovery periods, greater fat burning. But that has not always been the case.

Early studies correctly indicated that the oxidation of fat during muscle contraction was strictly aerobic in nature. That is, oxygen-related aerobic metabolism was the only known mechanism for breaking down and burning fat. Because steady state aerobic exercise – the most widely studied type of exercise - is literally defined by its elevated oxygen utilization, it was naturally assumed that longer duration lower intensity aerobic exercise was the best means of reducing body fat. Most fitness professionals are well aware of the so-called fat-burning zone of cardiovascular exercises that takes place with low to moderate intensity steady state exercise; this is indeed true. The aerobic argument makes further sense with the anecdotal acknowledgement that many endurance athletes are in fact thin.

As often occurs with the one-sided use of the scientific method of inquiry, this description was sound but evidence to the contrary was lacking. Put simply, exercise sciences' focus has and in many ways still lies with steady state and not cost per task analyses. Yet even without regard to overall energy costs, the scientific literature is now churning out confirmation that the use of intermittent exercise has the greatest impact on body weight and fat loss as compared to steady state aerobic exercise. The modernized explanation – fat fueling the afterburn periods of intermittent exercises – does indeed represent a rather radical departure from traditional aerobic, steady state, long distance running and cycling exercises that once dominated the body fat reduction mindset where, keep in mind, recovery costs are typically not considered. Times are changing.

A consensus has not yet been reached on why or how brief bouts of intermittent exercise create the physiological conditions and adaptations associated with fat loss. But there are certainly suggestions. As mentioned earlier, one straightforward example is that during recovery there is little to no muscular contraction providing ample conditions for fat oxidation. Another explanation is that due to the steady state mindset, the estimation of the caloric costs of intermittent exercise have been underestimated for years. Viewing intermittent stop-and-go exercise and recovery in the context of cost per task sets provides an alternative interpretation of the afterburn as a compilation of multiple recovery periods, not just one final afterburn when all is said and done.

Based on oxygen uptake measurements, the following energy cost conversions have been established (in fact, these have been known for well over a century). When glucose is the primary fuel of contracting muscle, every liter of oxygen consumed can be converted as 5.0 kcal:

Glucose oxidation: 1 liter of oxygen = 5.0 kcal

When fat is the primary fuel, for every liter of oxygen consumed, a conversion of 4.7 kcal is recognized:

Fat oxidation: 1 liter of oxygen = 4.7 kcal

Another interpretation is however apparent. Put another way, when glucose is used as fuel, for every kcal of energy, 0.20 liters of oxygen are consumed:

Glucose oxidation: 1 kcal = 0.20 liters of oxygen

With fat as a fuel, every kcal of energy requires the consumption of 0.21 liters of oxygen uptake:

Fat oxidation: 1 kcal = 0.21 liters of oxygen

Based on the above kcal-to-oxygen uptake perspective, 100 kcal of energy requires 20 liters of oxygen when using glucose as a fuel. With fat, that 100 kcal of energy requires 21 liters of oxygen.

When a measurement of oxygen consumption dictates energy costs, maximization occurs using fat as a fuel.

Applying this concept, 12 bouts of non-steady state intermittent exercise lasting 30 seconds each, with a recovery period after each bout lasting 2 minutes, would consist of 6 total minutes of exercise and 24 minutes of fat-burning recovery periods – 30 overall minutes. Doubling down, it's quite possible that a one hour stop-and-go workout may consist of 15 minutes or so of actual exercise, combined with 45 or so minutes of a collective afterburn. Considering fat as the preferred fuel, recovery would require more oxygen consumed as compared with the oxidation of glucose. Metabolic costs – that is, oxygen uptake - are elevated when fat is the primary fuel source. Of course, body composition changes in the form of reduced fat stores are also welcome.

Based on partial and impartial facts, I state this profoundly: any attempt to average together intermittent exercise and recovery periods into a single per minute estimate, simply follows steady state rules that dismiss the quantitative (increased oxygen uptake) and qualitative (increased fat burning) differences that the per task energy cost model promotes.

Exercise scientists and fitness professionals alike have all been trained to convert oxygen consumption into a kcal-related aerobic-narrative when attention should be placed on the exact opposite: based on energy (kcal) needs, the fuel being oxidized dictates the amount of oxygen consumed, not the other way around. Intermittent exercise and recovery periods need collective consideration where the appropriate kcal to oxygen uptake requirements for each are recognized.

If you are fortunate enough to have a diet and intermittent exercise program that decreases your body's fat stores, where does that fat go? The same holds true for all the lactic acid formed during the recruitment of faster twitch muscle fibers.

After giving a lecture on work and energy costs, I was informed by an audience member that she and her sister had each vowed to improve their lifestyle, with each subsequently losing a lot of weight in the process. "Where did it all go?" she asked, "my sister and I couldn't decide if all that fat disappeared as part of our poop or pee or perhaps we sweated it off...?"

"Nope" I replied, "it left with each and every one of your exhaled breaths."

She looked at me quite inquisitively, "no way".

Way.

Fat is a solid. It consists of carbon (C) and hydrogen (H) molecules and when considered in terms of the consumption of oxygen (O_2) and provision of its energy content, fat ends up in the format of two gases - carbon dioxide (CO_2) and water vapor (H_2O) - within your exhaled breath. Move and breathe!

Exercise programs designed to maximize caloric costs *and* fat loss should place a focus on recovery:

**The maximization of fat burning appears
to take place during those recovery periods
that follow intermittent exercise.**

If during each fat-burning recovery period, lower intensity physical movement is maintained – an active recovery - energy costs would be higher still. Keep moving, during both exercise <u>and</u> recovery.

VII.

HIIT Me: High Intensity Intermittent Training (Aerobic)

Higher intensity interval trainings (HIIT) first recorded appearance was in the latter 1930s with a pair of German physicians, Woldemar Gerschler and Herbert Randel. They had 'students' who smashed world records in the quarter and half-mile (400 and 800 meters) elongated sprints. There have been 2 or 3 more episodes of trending interest in HIIT since then - fads do indeed come and go. Yet some things remain the same. Higher intensity intermittent exercise is typically considered as a form of aerobic exercise with running and cycling serving as the primary formats. What's different is that while the exercise-type may be considered aerobic, it is not regarded as a prolonged steady state.

Studies have shown that at lower exercise intensities, exercise or work can continue to take place – muscular endurance - for hours on end. On the opposite end of the intensity spectrum, intermittent exercise performed near or at maximum levels also can occur for extended periods of time, but only when the work periods are brief (for example, seconds) and are coupled to an effective recovery period (for example, minutes). Performed in the "proper" exercise to recovery format, investigations of intermittent exercise have revealed a rather significant amount of work that can be completed utilizing a high intensity intermittent format. Quotation marks are applied around the word "proper" because the exercise to recovery ratio would likely differ between exercise types (aerobic vs. anaerobic for example) and among individuals (with for example, varying levels of fitness).

The Japanese exercise physiologist Izumi Tabata has triggered contemporary interest in intermittent exercise. But the story doesn't start with Professor Tabata. In fact, it was Irisawa Koichi, the head coach of the Japanese speed skating team. As with all great coaches, through empirical periods of trial and error, he pioneered the latest format of higher intensity intermittent training. Coach Koichi requested that his methods be scientifically tested and Professor Tabata responded accordingly.

Originally completed with bicycle ergometers, Tabata-training is the name now given to any and all brief, intense, periods of exercise and recovery that are coupled respectively in a 20-seconds on (exercise) and 10-seconds off (recovery) format that repeats itself 6 to 8 times. Four minutes are required for a complete Tabata routine, a downright agonizing four minutes if done correctly. While the fitness industry and its cohorts appear to have latched on to the machismo and bravado of the brief and intense protocol design, exercise scientists were treated to the first training format that resulted in *documented* gains of both (aerobic) oxygen uptake *and* (anaerobic) power output. In the realm of high intensity, both aerobic and anaerobic energy systems must be accounted for and it is most definitely possible to train for both simultaneously.

Before Tabata-training, increases in aerobic fitness were associated exclusively with aerobic exercise intensities, performed at some percentage of VO_2 max. Gains in anaerobic-related power output were thought to result specifically from sprint-type training, above and beyond VO_2 max (Tabata had subjects cycling at 170% of VO_2 max). While safety issues are unquestionably apparent, exercising briefly at or close to exhaustion can be a desired goal of a training routine and boy does it produce. But one must be in good physical condition before starting any higher intensity exercise routine – safety first. Begin gradually for example with lower intensity aerobic exercise, obtain a foundation-level of fitness and work your way up from there. Another downside exists with what I'll call sedentary recidivism: for many, high intensity exercise is not fun. And if you don't perceive exercise or activity as fun, you'll very likely stop doing it.

Recall the 4-minute carefully controlled Tabata routines previously described in the second chapter where moderately paced jump squats came in at 38 kcal and isotonic squats at 27 kcal. We also published the caloric costs of 3 all-out routines:

Maximum Effort Tabata Routine	Caloric Cost
Burpee and Lunge	69 kcal
Jump and push-up plyometrics	58 kcal
Squat & Dumbbell press resistance	42 kcal

And all-out means just that, a maximization of physical and perhaps psychological exertion. These could be considered decent energy cost numbers but I'm under the impression that in terms of maximizing caloric expenditure, energy cost numbers should not be in the double digits, but triple.

What about you? You undoubtedly know yourself best. With a focus on caloric cost, would you rather perform two intense all-out Tabata routines (8 minutes) at about 100-something kcals or, go for a 100 kcal, mile or so walk (20-25 minutes)? There is no wrong energy cost answer here. It's your choice.

The original Tabata routine was designed specifically, first and foremost, as a way to increase aerobic fitness *and* anaerobic power; that is, *performance*. It was not formulated with the intent of maximizing caloric costs or reducing body fat. From this perspective the original Tabata routine places primary value on the intense exercise periods and not on recovery. Yet again, this is not a book about the enhancement of physical performance. In terms of maximizing both caloric costs and especially fat burning periods, exercise programs may need to focus as much (if not more) on the recovery timetable. I don't have the data, but I speculate that in terms of maximizing the loss of body fat, a flipped Tabata routine might work better: with shorter exercise periods lasting 10 seconds and recovery periods of 20 seconds, or preferably longer.

Brief, intense, intermittent exercise bouts coupled with relatively longer recovery periods may help maximize both caloric costs and fat loss.

VIII.

Strongman: Heavy Load Intermittent Exercise (Anaerobic)

Perhaps no other type of exercise better displays the intermittent format of exercise and recovery as well as weight lifting or resistance training; typically, with the completion of a number of repetitions within a series of intermittent sets. Steady state aerobic exercise vernacular utilizes the term *intensity* to denote increases in steady rate power output. With anaerobic resistance training however, escalations in the amount of weight lifted are identified as an increase in *load*. Is it possible to equate the two: intensity and load, aerobic and anaerobic, respectively? You certainly cannot use the customary method of choice - the amount of oxygen consumed as an equivalent or standard - when aerobic exercise is receiving oxygen and anaerobic exercise may not.

A group of Portuguese exercise scientists under the tutelage of Victor Reis and Jose Vilaca-Alves recently attempted an oxygen-free comparison by creating a physiological match of lactic acid concentrations between steady state upper and lower body cycling exercises with upper body (bench press) and lower body (half squats) resistance exercises: intensity vs. load, respectively. Using similar blood lactic acid levels as a marker – a corresponding anaerobic threshold of sorts between the two - the anaerobic resistance training load was matched to a 'somewhat hard' to 'hard' steady state aerobic intensity (~67% of VO_2 max) at an astonishingly low 3% of a maximum lift for the half squat and 13% of a maximum lift for the bench press (that is, the percentage of a one repetition maximum lift or 1-RM).

If true, what a difference that match makes. Typical strength training programs rarely fall below a resistance of 60% of a maximum lift. Simply put, loads as low as 3 or 13% of maximum would not be called strength training by most weight lifters (a better term might be muscular endurance training).

Clearly, aerobic and anaerobic exercise need not be considered one and the same. Aerobic exercise is dependent on a continuous and large supply of oxygen. Within the brief sets of resistance exercise however, resides a minimal amount of exercise oxygen uptake. In fact, with lifting loads as low as 20% of a maximal voluntary contraction, blood flow to working skeletal muscle is compromised and so too is its oxygen supply. Fitness enthusiasts have capitalized on these conditions with a type of resistance training known as blood flow restriction (BFR) that has become quite popular worldwide, where a cuff of some type is placed at the top of the arms or thighs to further prevent or restrict blood flow. An interesting result from BFR training is that rather tremendous gains in arm and leg strength (performance) and muscle size (hypertrophy) have been recorded with lifting loads as low as 20% of a 1-RM.

Lifting low loads until you cannot lift them any longer - muscular failure - with *many* repetitions being the result, has also landed on the current weight lifting scene, producing strength and hypertrophy gains seen previously only with traditional heavier load lifting. In fact, after weeks of resistance training, cardiovascular (aerobic!) adaptations within muscle have been documented by lifting *any* load to the point of failure within a weight lifting set. Additional signs of changing times. Yet sadly (as seen before with isometric exercise), the energy costs do not appear to match the effort provided. Results of a pilot research project from our lab have shown that squatting a weight at 50% of a 1-RM, to muscular failure for 3 consecutive sets, with 90 seconds of recovery between sets, followed by a ~15 minute final afterburn period, resulted in an averaged caloric cost of about 50 kcal for women and 70 kcal for men (roughly 50 to 70 repetitions overall). These results mimic the energy costs of all-out Tabata-type training.

Resistance training programs designed to increase performance may not necessarily maximize overall energy costs.

But all is not lost. What is unique and helpful to the maximization of resistance training energy costs is that after a standard weight lifting set has ended, oxygen uptake may continue to climb, *peaking in recovery* and not during the actual resistance exercise period. To the contrary, with the steady state model, oxygen uptake peaks during exercise and *always falls* throughout recovery.

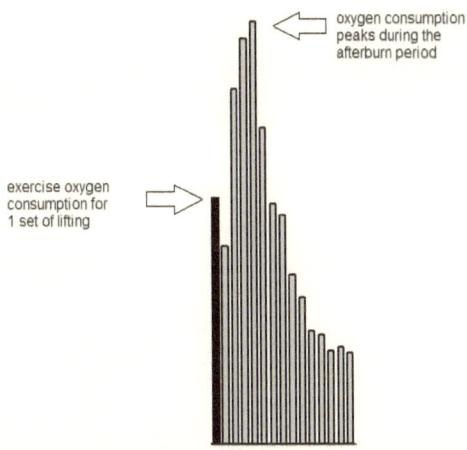

oxygen consumption
peaks during the
afterburn period

exercise oxygen
consumption for
1 set of lifting

Each vertical bar in the above figure demonstrates a 15 second measurement of oxygen uptake. The first black bar represents a 15 second period of weight lifting, followed by 4 minutes of recovery. Note that for resistance exercise, oxygen uptake peaks in recovery not during the exercise period – this pattern was seen when the weight lifted was at least 60% of a 1-RM lift. According to oxygen uptake measurements, the greatest caloric cost comes not during the resistance training exercise, but in the recovery.

Why the difference… why does recovery oxygen uptake fall after aerobic exercise but continue to climb after high-load anaerobic resistance exercise? The likely answer is that under extreme energy demand conditions (high load) and especially when oxygen delivery is compromised, contracting muscle uses a storage of anaerobic energy in the form of two high energy phosphates: 1) adenosine tri-phosphate or ATP and, 2) creatine phosphate or phospho-creatine (PCr). These limited high energy stores can only supply energy for a few to several seconds, and as they approach depletion a muscle's ability to contract falters. With resistance exercise, moderate to heavy loads prevent blood flow to and from working muscle and the production of lactic acid is a given. Under last resort conditions, resistance exercise relies on the use of the high energy phosphates to fuel muscle contraction and afterwards, it appears critical for restoration of these high energy molecules to promptly take place. The moment the weight being lifted is racked, muscular forces are terminated and oxygen delivery resumes. That oxygen is straightaway utilized to re-store a muscles high energy phosphate content back to initial levels and the result is a spike in recovery oxygen consumption (the energy held within fat and lactic acid molecules fuels ATP and PCr restoration).

So how is resistance exercise currently modeled in terms of energy costs? By recognizing exercise science history and its steady state aerobic origins, the answer may not be too surprising. A brief bout of resistance exercise, say a 30 second set of weight lifting, is typically followed by a recovery period that may last a few minutes, Then, more sets are completed with recovery periods following each and every set. Under steady state consideration, only when you get to the last set is that final recovery considered an excess post-exercise oxygen consumption (EPOC) or afterburn period.

Using this traditional precedent, all of the previous resistance exercise and recovery components are averaged into a single caloric cost per minute estimate: all resistance exercise and recovery periods – except for that final afterburn – are considered as one. This model has been applied to resistance exercise not because it's the correct thing to do, but because right or wrong the steady state model currently characterizes most published energy cost estimates of exercise and physical activity – it's currently the only thing to do. The next figure reveals this methodology.

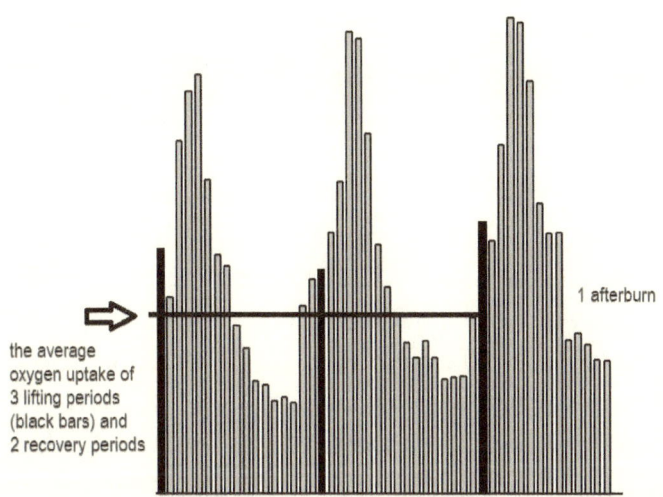

the average
oxygen uptake of
3 lifting periods
(black bars) and
2 recovery periods

1 afterburn

As applied to intermittent exercise, the steady state per minute method averages the three 15 second weight lifting periods (black vertical bars) with the two 4-minute recovery periods following the first and second set (vertical gray bars) to obtain a single per minute energy cost estimate; only after the third and last set is completed is recovery oxygen uptake considered to be an afterburn period (also known as excess post-exercise oxygen consumption, EPOC).

When modeling the energy costs of exercise in any form, steady state methodology still rules. Even the most careless analysis of the 2 previous figures reveals a clear roller coaster pattern of measured oxygen uptake throughout both exercise and recovery. In no way shape or form does this up-and-down pattern provide steady state justification. Yet based on standard practice, most exercise scientists continue to take the oxygen uptake peaks and valleys of resistance exercise and average them into a single per minute steady state interpretation. Lather. Rinse. Repeat. Indeed.

Our Exercise Science Laboratory has created a different

approach to intermittent resistance exercise in terms of a cost per task estimate, not an averaged steady state cost per minute. By treating exercise and recovery periods as separate entities new interpretations can be realized. As an example, two former students compared *equivalent* work <u>and</u> *equivalent* recovery periods between two resistance exercise formats: lifting the same weight (the bench press exercise at 65% of 1-RM) for 2 sets of 8 repetitions followed respectively by 2 recovery periods (3.5 minutes of rest between each set) as compared to 8 sets of 2 repetitions, each set being followed by 8 respective recovery periods (30 seconds rest between sets for a total of 3.5 minutes). Here's what the oxygen uptake numbers looked like:

	2 sets – 8 reps	8 sets – 2 reps
Oxygen consumption	1.8 liters	2.6 liters

Acknowledging fat-burning as an aerobic oxygen consuming endeavor, based on the above numbers, increasing the number of exercise and recovery periods also increases overall oxygen uptake. From a cost per task perspective, accumulating exercise and intermittent recovery periods creates a likely scenario for a greater oxidation of fat (when the anaerobic costs were included with the oxygen uptake data shown above, the overall costs were actually the same for each protocol at 15 kcal).

Mainstream descriptions of resistance training program design are exemplified in a trilogy format: **1)** the load lifted as percentage of a one repetition maximum lift (% 1-RM), **2)** the number of repetitions completed, and **3)** the number of sets performed. We certainly identify with this design but have taken the additional step of applying each of these 3 measures in terms of work performed, with work being the product of the amount of weight lifted and the upward vertical distance force is applied. Our ability to quantify resistance exercise work allowed us to obtain a measure of not only the overall costs but also the work-to-cost efficiency and that data specifically revealed exactly where the highest energy costs are along the strength training (high load) and muscular endurance training (lower load) spectrum.

Using the bench press exercise we had subjects perform two consecutive sets at 3 different loads with muscular failure defining the end of each set. The next table identifies both total energy costs and efficiency for each load, with efficiency recognized as a unit of work (Joules) per energy cost (kcal) – efficiency is best with muscular endurance-type training:

Two Consecutive Sets of Bench Press: Lifting to Failure for both Sets

%1-RM	Total Cost (kcal)	Work (J)	Joules per kcal (J·kcal⁻¹)	Repetitions
70%	23	637	28	22
80%	22	512	23	16
90%	17	325	19	9

For two sets of resistance training, a heavier load (90% 1-RM) results in less work completed (325 Joules) at a lower total energy cost (17 kcal), but it also represents the most inefficient of the three loads at 19 Joules of work per kcal of energy cost. At the lowest load - 70% of 1RM - the most work is completed (637 Joules) at the highest cost (23 kcal). Efficiency however, is much improved at the lowest load: 28 Joules of work per kcal spent. This trend also was found for lifts that were not completed to failure.

From an efficiency point of view, if the 90% 1-RM protocol was completed twice (4 sets overall), the amount of work compared to two sets of the 70% 1-RM protocol would almost be equivalent, increasing by 2%, but the total costs would increase by 32%. In the context of inefficiency, multiple brief intermittent high load lifting periods or sets, each followed with a recovery, helps maximize energy costs. Endless repetitions are not the answer.

Here's a shocking example of how an increased repetition number and an outrageously high perceived exertion need not be associated with maximal energy costs: Remember the blood flow restriction (BFR) training method previously mentioned? At 50% of a 1-RM for the squat exercise, our most impressive subject "burned" an overall 110 kcal. Not bad, you might think, but there are caveats: hoisting 195 pounds, the first set consisted of 52 repetitions (followed by a 90 second recovery), the second set lasted all of 7 reps (followed by a 90 second recovery) with the third and final set completed with 5 additional repetitions (followed by a 15-minute supine recovery): 23 overall minutes. The work to cost ratio was 25 Joules per kcal, both a mediocre efficiency and inefficiency estimate. Here's some additional background information. Completing this identical protocol, we had one subject complain of nausea, another actually "tossed cookies" after it was all over, one guy couldn't stand for a full 5 minutes afterward and, I kid you not, yet another momentarily lost consciousness (911 was called and all ended well for everyone involved). How does a 100 kcal, 23-minute walk sound now?

We need to get real here, training for performance and training to maximize energy costs can in fact be mutually exclusive. Endless repetitions of exercise can have a negative influence on enjoyment and from the standpoint of efficiency they don't necessarily maximize energy costs either. As stated within the first paragraph of this text, perhaps a majority of available information suggests weight loss is far better achieved by diet and not exercise. I still agree with that.

Another potential benefit of using brief (low repetitions) and multiple sets to better escalate costs is seen in the next figure, where the recovery energy cost component grows larger with each successive set as the anaerobic cost simultaneously becomes smaller. This figure demonstrates the growing fat burning capabilities of repeated bouts of recovery as attached to repeated intermittent sets of resistance exercise.

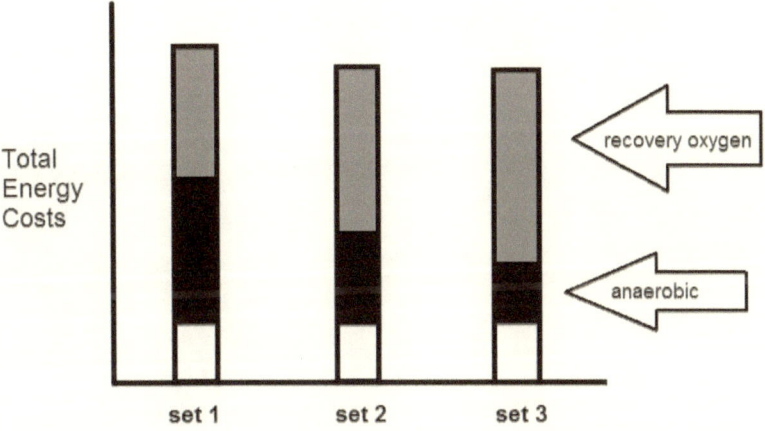

Three metabolic characteristics of three sets of the bench press exercise are shown above (70% of 1-RM, 5 repetitions per set; this was not a difficult workload): 1) the top grey bars represents the amount of kcal provided by the volume of oxygen consumed in the recovery (afterburn) of each set, 2) the middle black bars indicate the anaerobic energy cost (dictated by lactic acid levels following each set), and 3) the bottom white bars represent the amount of oxygen consumed during each set. Note that as more sets are completed the volume of recovery oxygen consumption grows larger as anaerobic costs shrink in comparison. With less anaerobic lactic acid production, the stage is set for an increased oxidation of fat with increasing sets (as the high energy phosphates are restored). This trend also has been seen with repeated brief intermittent bouts of aerobic exercise (for example, sprinting and cycling).

In addition to weight lifting experience, heavier loads and/
or lifting to muscular failure requires direct supervision by a
personal trainer or a capable workout partner.

This chapters take home message:

**Brief intermittent heavy load sets, each coupled to
a relatively extended recovery period, appears to
better maximize energy costs and fat burning:
fewer repetitions, more sets.**

IX.

Think Big: Large Muscle Groups

**The larger the working muscle mass
the greater the caloric cost.**

Contrary to previous chapters this take home message has been provided up-front, as an absolute given. Whether movement consists only of your body's mass or the inclusion of a dumbbell or barbell or any other type of weight or resistance, increasing the amount of working muscle maximizes costs.

We found that for *equivalently measured work* performed among the bench press, the squat and the deadlift exercises, energy costs were lowest for the bench press, highest for the deadlift and in-between for the squat – these were cost per set estimates. For our investigation, experienced lifters chose a weight not based on a percentage of a 1-repetition maximum (% 1-RM), but instead as a random selection with instructions to lift the weight until a perceived exertion of 'somewhat hard to hard' was reached. Low weight many reps, more weight less reps, our

analyses had it all and perhaps most importantly we had a measure of work as well.

Roughly translated, the energy requirements of curling a
20-pound weight a distance of ½ meter, 10-times, with your
right biceps muscle would enact a specific caloric cost. Lift the
exact same 20 pounds with 2 arms (right and left biceps, a
larger muscle mass) and the cost should increase. Done again,
the identical workload with the bench press exercise (arms,
chest, and shoulders) the cost would be higher still. Equivalent
work using the squat exercise (more muscle) would result in,
you guessed it, an even higher energy cost. All at an equivalent
work load.

As an explanation: with your right hand you may be capable
of handgrip exercise producing 20 pounds of pressure, but the
use of such a small muscle mass would not be all that costly;
apply the same 20-pounds with a two-legged leg press and the
costs would be significantly greater. Of course, the 5 digits on
your right hand weigh far less than your two legs, and those
extra forces involved with the displacement of the heavier limbs
of your lower body helps explain why energy costs are greater.

You don't in fact need to lift an external load. Your body's
mass is everything you've got and moving it all – up and down
and from here to there - can certainly be costly, no equipment
needed. Think whole-body calisthenics for example burpees
and hip-hop dance... move bigly!

While on the subject of dance, we also need another cry-
out to plyometrics – leaping, jumping, bounding and the like.
Recall that the forces of inertia require the recruitment of larger
muscle masses, increasing overall energy costs. But be careful,
whether deserved or not, plyometric exercise routines have a
nasty reputation in terms of injury promotion and should only

be performed by those who would already consider themselves in good to great physical condition.

Energy costs are maximized along with the extent of whole body movement – perform identical tasks with more muscles and caloric costs are maximized.

X.

The Price of Pain: Muscle Failure

Muscular failure has the effect of making resistance exercise and recovery energy costs more expensive. When lifting a weight until it can be lifted no longer, we found a somewhat specific 5.0 kcal additional cost (per set) for any given comparison between *equivalent* bench press work performed under non-failure conditions – again, these estimates were completed per task or set. This is unlikely to be true for other resistance exercises, as larger and smaller working muscle masses would likely have larger and smaller (respectively) added costs that are associated with lifting a weight. As a hypothetical example, the squat exercise uses a much larger muscle mass as compared to the bench press so that lifting to fatigue may result in, perhaps, an extra 10 kcals or so per set as opposed to 5 kcal.

While no means a large absolute number, from a relative perspective the 5 kcal increase that lifting to muscular failure promoted for 1-set of the bench press exercise was an incredible 56% greater as compared to equivalent work where failure does not take place. Interpretation is everything. Again, it's critical to establish that muscular failure occurred at an *equivalent work-load* as compared to non-failure lifting – no additional work is being completed under either condition.

Compare two identical twins at an equivalent body weight. One twin can only do 10 push-ups before collapsing in fatigue; the second can do 50 push-ups if she wanted, but was asked to stop at ten. The amount of work completed would be the same for each twin (10 push-ups) but the additional energy cost would be ~5.0 kcal greater with the twin who reached muscular failure. If the first twin trains faithfully for a few weeks, imagine her new accomplishment might be 20 pushups until exhaustion set in. Compared to the second twin's 20 easily-performed pushups, the same 5.0 kcal increase would be seen with the first twin who worked until failure. And so on, a relatively stable increase in fatigue-related caloric expenditure, regardless of the amount of pushups (work) completed.

From the perspective of efficiency, non-failure conditions resulted in the performance of 32 Joules of bench press work per kcal of energy cost; muscular failure lowered that to 14 Joules of work per kcal spent. Lifting a weight to failure is more inefficient and maximizes energy costs.

So what causes a muscle to reach the point where force production fails? A professor of mine long ago put it best, "fatigue is a very complex subject". He was correct then and he's correct now. From a 2-dimensional standpoint the *depletion* of something, say oxygen or fuel (glucose or high energy phosphates) can cause fatigue. On the other hand, an *accumulation* of a myriad of metabolic by-products – such as lactic acid - within muscle may also impair contractile force. And that's without mention of all the myriad of happenstance in-between. In fact, fatigue is thought by some academics to originate within your nervous system, not within muscle. The subject matter is indeed multifaceted.

We spend a bit of time in my exercise physiology classes talking about lactic acid with 9 or 10 out of every 10 students convinced, before any discussion on the subject begins, that an accumulation of lactic acid is the chief culprit in the fatigue process. One metaphor I use to describe this prejudice is that of a fight breaking out within a crowd. The police show up and randomly grab one constituent out of the ensuing violence, throw them to the ground and upon arrest demand to know, "Hey lactic acid! Why did you start this mess?"

It doesn't end well for my students either. Over the course of days and weeks I promote lactate as only one of many possible fatigue factors. In the simplest of terms lactic acid is, after all, a single molecule of glucose that has been split into two halves: 2 molecules of lactic acid. As mentioned earlier, muscle actually burns this stuff as fuel, just like glucose and fat. Yet at the end of the lesson, when again asked for a show of hands to answer the following, "name a chief instigator in the fatigue process?", 8 or 9 out of 10 continue to reply, lactic acid. The grip of bias is a tight one. But to be fair, exercise scientists themselves are still very much divided on whether lactic acid does, does not or to what extent it may or may not, cause rather than promote, fatigue.

Final word: **Exercising to muscular failure maximizes overall exercise costs**. Yet dependent on personality, failure can hurt and the emotional response can be reactionary: failure equals quit. Be careful with exercise formats that influence both the body and the psyche and not always in a positive way. Remember also that the primary guidelines presented within this text are to maximize costs, not physical prowess.

XI.

Do It for Health

A few bursts of intense exercise sprinkled throughout the week can promote a number of things: increased physical performance, a maximization of energy expenditure, the burning of body fat, and as this chapter describes, significant improvements in health. Yet the potential risks involved by periodically and dramatically increasing your metabolic rate must undergo serious consideration. Couch-potato or not, all should submit to periodic health screening and health provider clearance, then gradually and steadily work their way toward a more respectable level of fitness. Workouts demanding strength, speed and high power output are quite literally not for the faint of heart. The achievement of a foundation of fitness provides the best starting point before the initiation of advanced exercise intensities and/or loads.

Human movement requires physical activity, defined by the American Heritage dictionary as, "the state of being active; energetic action or movement; liveliness". Activity is then, physical movement that happens. Clearly, under this definition, knitting, card playing and basket weaving can be considered forms of physical activity, but for the sake of this discussion, activity will be interpreted in a larger and more physical context like, gardening, washing a car, and walking the dog. Any and all types of manual labor works. Pushing a lawn mower counts, riding one does not.

The word 'exercise' has been defined in several contexts, one of them being, "an activity having a specified aspect." In this regard exercise is anticipated, planned and organized. The American College of Sports Medicine (ACSM) guidelines serve as a wonderful example. Cardiorespiratory fitness is achieved, we are instructed, via aerobic exercise performed: with large muscle masses moving rhythmically and continuously, 3-5 days per week, at an intensity of 30% to 59% of heart rate reserve for 30 to 60 minutes per day. You can't get much more planned and organized than that. ACSM guidelines have been conveniently developed from and specifically for a rather large variety of populations, healthy or not, exercise *is* medicine according to the ACSM and needs to be prescribed accordingly.

The author of this text put himself through school at a time when "exercise" was defined strictly in an aerobic context. The words, "put himself through school" suggest some sort of physical activity took place. The words 'labor union' better describe the ordeal and the day was not done when the labor ended. After a day of jackhammering through concrete or digging ditches through dirt and rock, aerobic exercise still needed to be completed because, as I was taught, the achievement of health dictated strict aerobic rules of engagement; intermittent physical activity and labor in-and-of itself was not thought to promote health.

More disparaging news indicated that steady state exercise

was not the cure-all it was once suggested to be. Not too long ago fitness zealots erroneously proclaimed that hard-core exercise training, for example running marathons, could actually eradicate heart disease. This idea was hit hard with the death of Jim Fixx, author of the wildly successful book, "The Complete Book of Running". Like many others, he died doing just that. Disease is both inherited and of self-creation and for many of us it is a convoluted amalgamation of both. Heart disease risk is identified as a compilation of risk factors, and with underlying disease being present, a dramatic rise in metabolism most assuredly has the potential to trigger a cardiac event. Even so, regular exercise and physical activity <u>both</u> go a long way in the promotion of health and well-being.

Of course nutrition plays a role. While it is generally thought that people who eat more calories than they expend gain weight, it's also plausible that some are born with a metabolism that prefers one substrate over another. Blessed are those "fat burners" among us who throughout a day burn fat as a fuel – they eat fat, they burn fat. Less fortunate are those "glucose burners" who tend to do just that, while retaining and storing the fat they eat. True or not, there's more to the story. We assume, of course, that exercise helps us lose weight. Yet exercise may have more influence on weight gain. A recent study concluded that the number of Americans who don't exercise or engage in meaningful physical activity on a regular basis has more than doubled in women and more than tripled in men over the past twenty years. Over the same period caloric intake hasn't changed that much, yet body weight relentlessly continues to climb. The take home interpretation:

Today's diet promotes tomorrow's weight loss or gain; exercise and activity habits are more likely to affect life-long weight gain.

In fact, *most* people are overweight because of behaviors reflected by the environment in which they live and not because of a poor or ineffective metabolism. Within a society where processed meals high in sugar and fat are often the norm, weight gain over time for many of us is a given. Living under such circumstances, the goal of weight loss should be nutritional - reducing the sugars, fats and perhaps most importantly the preparation of our meals. Current mainstream guidelines –interpretations you can take or leave – suggest the less "processed" our foods the better. Consider the characteristic grocery store with fresh produce present at the stores four walled perimeters, and most boxed, canned and plasticized processed foods found within the aisles. You're better off purchasing from the stores outskirts.

I'm asked quite often about what people should do to lose weight and while an exercise physiologist by training my thoughts on weight loss focus on eating, at least for our short term day-to-day existence. A top 10 list would focus on thinking about how much and what type of food is being consumed along with the behaviors associated with why you're eating, what format that food was purchased in (raw versus packaged, for example), where you bought it (groceries vs. fast food), how that food was prepared (e.g., fried vs. baked), why you are eating (daily dinner vs. tailgate party) - stuff like that. Again, diet is likely the most important aspect of short term weight gain and loss. Eight, nine and ten on that list would focus on the design of appropriate exercise and recovery programs.

Here's a shocking example of an interpretational about-face: saturated fat consumption has been heavily promoted over the years as a major health related risk factor in the onset of heart disease, while at the same time the roles of sugars and refined carbohydrates appears to have been very much underestimated. The consequences of such pronouncement can be frightening.

High carbohydrate - low fat diets as recommended by the American Heart Association (AHA) among others, have the potential to elevate blood sugar and insulin levels, both of which may represent a greater risk factor than saturated fat intake. As crazy as it may sound, those *authorities* responsible for the very creation of public health policy dietary guidelines – lower fat, higher carbohydrate - now suggest that a contributory or causal (!) relationship may have been introduced with the creation of said guidelines. That is, an up-tick in obesity and diabetes, each occur at about the same time as the universal introduction of high carb/low fat diets for all. Crazy indeed.

From the standpoint of physical movement, brief intense intermittent exercise has been well demonstrated to have a favorable impact on your carbohydrate-related health. And by brief, I mean brief. Professor Martin Gibala's research group at McMaster University in Canada has shown that as little as 3 sets of 20 seconds of all-out bicycle sprints (1 full minute) performed three times per week (3 minutes overall) achieved similar health improvement as compared to the completion of moderate intensity aerobic bicycling performed for 45 minutes three times per week (that's 2 hours and 15 minutes overall). Why is this?

It was earlier mentioned that oxygen was dangerous stuff, so too is the sugar within the processed food you eat and goodness-grief we certainly need both of these to survive. Under normal conditions your nervous system for example feasts exclusively on glucose as a fuel. The danger comes it appears, when relatively higher levels of glucose are continuously and regularly circulating throughout your blood stream, a result of the steady consumption of processed food. High blood glucose and insulin levels damage blood vessels, and that cardiovascular harm seemingly outweighs high circulating fat levels. Within your blood stream greater levels of glucose are the enemy, not fat.

As mentioned earlier, intense exercise rapidly consumes glucose molecules stored within glycogen, and those glycogen stores are subsequently replenished by that glucose found within the blood stream: simply put, regular exercise and physical activity help remove excess glucose from your bloodstream. Continuous glucose/glycogen turnover is actually good for your heart and blood vessels and high intensity intermittent training (HIIT) may best achieve this effect.

Remember the 150 kcal daily caloric cost minimum mentioned in this text's Introduction? That's the number of calories thought to be required when health benefits begin to accrue – 1000 kcals of *aerobic steady state exercise* per week. I haven't made the measurement, but it's highly unlikely that 3 minutes of high intensity intermittent cycling per week is associated with 1000 kcals of overall energy costs – that's more than 300 kcal for a single minute of exercise plus recovery! My goodness, we are now leaving the heat production rates of biological metabolism and approaching that of combustion. Actually that interpretation is one of complete exaggeration. Channeling my educated-guess powers to the best of my ability, I doubt a single minute of all-out intermittent cycling for most of us comes remotely close to approaching 100 kcal – perhaps 30 - 40 kcal? If so, we have yet another difference between steady state exercise, intermittent exercise, and their associated health-related cost-to-benefit ratios. A caloric count of 150 kcal per day for steady state exercise may indeed be an appropriate boundary for health improvement; for high intensity intermittent exercise however it appears way less than that.

Lowering blood glucose levels – not necessarily reducing fat consumption – subsequently reduces health risk, especially that of heart disease.

As with health improvement, the choice of an exercise design with a focus on weight loss is most certainly subjective. But 50 calories a day of movement translates to the requirement of 80 days to lose a pound of fat (4000 kcal); 150 kcals a day of physical activity would require almost 27 days. Recognizing that choices are personal, a goal of about 1 pound of fat loss every 10 days sounds somewhat reasonable. That equates to 400 kcal of movement - every single day. In truth, within the society in which I live, I would consider that a lot to ask of the masses.

To summarize, regular physical activity, aerobic steady state exercise, and intermittent higher intensity exercise all have the potential, to varying degrees, of tapping into a working muscle's glycogen stores that are restored by subsequently removing circulating glucose within the blood stream, lowering blood sugar levels in the process.

So what type of exercise or activity program works best for you? There's only one way to find out: give them all a try and invest in a good professional trainer who can provide ample guidance and motivation. Higher intensity intermittent exercise doesn't have to be an all-the-time thing, just an as-often-as-you-please thing or perhaps you may find it's a not-my-cup-of-tea thing.

Again, the starting part is movement, regardless of the format. Active or athlete, steady state or not, high intensity or low, in terms of health related issues, both regular physical activity and exercise promote your overall well-being. Discussion over. Drop mic. Exit.

Choose that type of physical movement you enjoy most, do it regularly and health benefits are sure to follow.

XII.

An Exercise Science Lab

My students and I, of course, have used all the standard tools of a typical Exercise Science Lab: a metabolic cart for the measurement of oxygen and carbon dioxide, blood lactic acid analyzers, cycle ergometers, treadmills, spirometers, ECG recorders, heart rate monitors, body fat analyzers, sphygmomanometers…etc. What makes us different however is that we have the ability to measure work during resistance exercise and that has had a rather profound impact on our data interpretation. Just as importantly, we view exercise and recovery as being very much different from one another, with separate oxygen consumption to kcal conversions for each: exercise periods in terms of glucose oxidation and recovery periods from the perspective of fat oxidation. Anaerobic energy costs are also considered.

At first glance lifting a weight appears to be pretty one dimensional – you pick it up, you put it down. However, that movement can be much more 3-dimensional than realized. Of course there is the up-and-down undertaking of the lift itself. But the weight's movement also must be balanced, producing ever-so-slightly back-and-forth and side-to-side motion, influencing force production as well as its estimated costs. You also are very likely to slightly vary the vertical distance the weight travels for each and every repetition within a given set. What we needed was a device that could, with validity, accurately and precisely measure the distance a given weight was lifted, while keeping all other movements to a minimum - we needed to better control and quantify work in terms of weight lifted and the displacement of the bar.

A Smith Machine served our purpose as a horizontal bar moving along fixed tracks allows lifting only in an upward and downward vertical plane. Faculty and students from the School of Engineering were subsequently asked to modify our Smith Machine so we could obtain a measure of work. This resulted in a bit of a dilemma. Work is typically expressed in terms of an upward movement, perpendicular from Earth's surface. To the contrary, lowering that same weight to the original starting position dismisses any work that was accomplished. Our engineers first shared with us their comedic skills. I was told that they would be painting a large "0" on cardboard and hanging it from the back of the Smith machine as a recording of work performed. Lift a weight upward and work took place, lower the weight to the starting position and work was re-set to zero. In effect no work takes place when lifting *and* lowering a weight.

LOL!

I thought about getting them all pocket-protectors for their birthdays.

Yet this group had other talents. Like us, they too have a Senior Thesis class where clients come in with problems that teams of undergraduate student engineers compete to solve. The winning design for our project was a simple flywheel that turns a mechanical signal into an electrical one as the weight lifting bar moves upward (downward movement was discarded). We track movement in millimeters (actually, slightly less than a millimeter).

While somewhat unique, our device does not account for inertia; the overcoming of a mass's acceleration towards earth. All weight lifted is in fact constantly being pulled toward earth with an acceleration of 9.8 meters per second^2. Note the power sign. In order to overcome that acceleration, a supplementary force must be applied in addition to that associated directly with the vertical lifting of a specific weight. We do not account for inertia in our work model, but we can account for the amount of weight lifted and the vertical distance the lifting bar travels. This is how work is defined, as Joules (J), within our lab:

$$\text{Work (J)} = \text{weight lifted} \times \text{vertical distance}$$

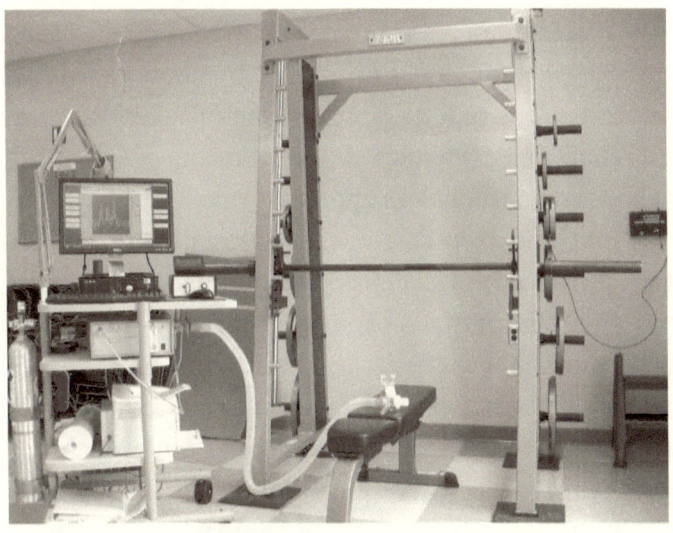

Our Smith weight lifting machine. Also shown at left is the metabolic cart (with PC) and air collection hose and mouthpiece. At right, mounted on the wall, is the electrical readout of resistance training work.

Carefully tracking the Smith Machine's bar movement for a very specific 1 meter of vertical displacement revealed a co-efficient of variation (CV) for a single up-and-down lift (1 repetition) of 0.25%. Among sets of ten repetitions, 1-meter lift each, vertical movements generated a 0.75% variation. The co-efficient of variability describes just that, variation or error. So our device, whether per rep or per set, has less than 1% measurement error, an absolutely acceptable number.

In terms of the actual lifting of a weight for multiple repetitions by an experienced weight lifter, the co-efficient of variation for bar movement was about 5%, indicating a noticeable but acceptable variation for each repetition completed. Again, no back-and-forth or side-to-side motion happens with the Smith Machine. The majority of the up-and-down variability comes from the lifter who unknowingly alters the vertical displacement themselves, from start (bottom) to finish (top).

Valid measurements are an absolute requirement of any scientific investigation so you might imagine how elated I was in terms of what our modified Smith Machine could accomplish with a reliable measurement of work. Lifting a weight freely – dumbbells and barbells - as opposed to along the fixed track of a Smith machine likely creates energy cost differences between the two in that the associated costs to maintain balance are not a part of the Smith machine. There may very well be further energy cost differences between a Smith Machine exercise and its free weight version. But I'll take the cost-to-benefit trade-off here (for the moment) and stick with our Smith Machine.

Unfortunately, our modified Smith Machine further created a limitation so huge that our findings could be rendered useless in terms of practical application – the unit measured is foreign to most of us. Work is measured in a unit known as the Joule. Yet most every resistance training conversation within most fitness facilities the world over is dictated by a load (in pounds or kilograms) taken as a percent of a one repetition maximum (%1-RM) with an amount of work recognized by the number of repetitions and sets completed. That language is weight, reps, sets. Weight lifting or resistance training is not designated in the context of Joules. I doubt that within my life-time, within any gymnasium, the language will switch over to, "Hey, how many Joules was your workout?" "Ha, my Joules are bigger than yours!" I'll stop there.

Yet from the scientific necessity of validity, a reasonable analyses of energy costs that are associated with a specific amount of work can now be obtained, and I'll take that payoff too, Joules and all. With these estimates in hand we began to look at things in a different way, not only in terms of the total costs but also in terms of efficiency. Make no mistake, if you want to maximize energy costs you have to minimize efficiency, and as mentioned earlier we can now estimate that too.

Our per task or per set, 3 components, total energy cost estimate is converted from the following measures:

1. Exercise oxygen uptake (assuming glucose oxidation)
2. Recovery oxygen uptake (assuming fat oxidation)
3. Blood lactic acid levels

We decided to begin our focus on single sets of submax-imal lifting as we did not want muscular failure or fatigue to interfere with our energy cost estimates. In addition, lifting movements were standardized at a cadence of 1.5 seconds up and 1.5 seconds down; 3 seconds per repetition, so as to mini-mize the potential impact of slower and faster lifting speeds on the energy cost outcome. For each and every resistance exercise study we have conducted to date, what was found was rather eye-opening. From a per set or multiple set perspective:

1. Oxygen related energy costs during resistance exercise represented the *lowest* overall cost.
2. Recovery oxygen uptake represented the *highest* overall cost.
3. Anaerobic energy costs could be as high as recovery (or almost as high).

As compared to per minute aerobic steady state exercise, our cost per set findings were indeed startling. They are in fact completely opposite the steady state model where: 1) exercise oxygen uptake measurements always dominate, 2) recovery oxygen consumption can be ignored or questioned in terms of being a significant contributor to the overall energy cost, and 3) anaerobic energy costs do not undergo representation.

Unlearn and re-learn once again. It's time to spread the word.

For all of our investigations to date, exercise and recovery oxygen uptake in addition to blood lactate levels, when converted into an energy cost estimate, all increase in a perfectly predictable manner as compared with the amount of work completed. Moreover, we can now present an amended energy cost analysis that includes work-to-cost efficiency.

Let's re-visit the application of a work-to-cost efficiency estimation. The next table identifies not only the overall energy cost for single sets of resistance exercise, but also the energy cost per volume or amount of work performed. We're searching for inefficiency here – the least bang for the buck - and it can be seen below in terms of Joules of work per kcal of energy cost ($J \cdot kcal^{-1}$):

Cost, Work and Inefficiency of the Bench Press: Lifting to Muscular Failure (1 set)

%1-RM	Reps	Total Cost (kcal)	Work (J)	Joules per kcal (J·kcal⁻¹)	Time (seconds)
37%	36	15	514	34	108
46%	25	14	439	31	75
56%	20	14	426	30	60
70%	12	12	342	28	36
80%	11	11	274	25	24
90%	8	8	167	21	12

From a maximizing energy cost perspective, a knee jerk interpretation of the above table might be to focus on that workload that promoted the greatest overall or total cost. At a load of 37% of a 1-Repetition Maximum (RM), it took an average of 36 repetitions to reach muscular failure and 108 seconds to complete that task at a total cost of 15 kcal. When searching for inefficiency it was the largest load - at 90% of a 1-RM - that had the least amount of work completed per kcal of energy cost: 21 Joules of work per 1 kcal (at a total cost of 8 kcal). Compare that to the muscular endurance workload where for every kcal utilized, 34 Joules of work were completed. From the perspective of efficiency, the least bang for your buck in terms of work-performed-per-kcal-of-energy-cost comes not with muscular endurance-type training, but instead with the highest and briefest workloads. This identical work-to-energy-cost pattern also described submaximal bench press lifts where muscular failure was not the end result: 7 reps at 36 Joules·kcal⁻¹, 14 reps at 37 Joules·kcal⁻¹, and 21 reps at 39 Joules·kcal⁻¹.

Most assuredly muscular endurance training comes at a cost. Yet if total energy costs are matched by the amount of work completed, at an overall cost of 15 kcal, just 2 sets of lifting at 90% of 1-RM (a total of 8 reps in 24 seconds) are needed to equal the caloric expenditure of 1 set of 36 reps at 37% of 1-RM (1.8 minutes).

Want to maximize the energy costs of resistance training? Lots of brief sets using heavy loads appears to be the answer; and don't forget about the requisite multiple recovery periods that follow.

If you further pursue resistance exercise program design from the perspectives of both inefficiency and time, at an identical muscular endurance work time of 108 seconds (15 overall kcal) you could perform 9 intermittent sets at 90% of a 1-RM, at a total cost of 72 kcals – that's quite a maximization. Consider also the additional expenses of active recovery periods between sets (move!), involving as little as 'walking around' for a few to several minutes before the next set and not passively lying, sitting, or standing.

As new answers came, so too did new problems. Going back to the Muscle Failure chapter, the condition of muscular failure (1 set) resulted in an energy cost efficiency of 14 Joules of work per kcal of energy cost, yet the lifting-to-failure table presented in this chapter does not approach that level of inefficiency at 21 Joules·kcal^{-1}. Why is this? The answer, as always, is in the analysis and interpretation.

As previously detailed, scientists sometimes search for relationships by forcing a straight line through what can at times be disparate data points. Linearity you may recall lies at the heart of the steady state perspective. And make no mistake about this, our total energy cost model also reveals a perfectly predictable linear relationship between work and its associated aerobic and anaerobic exercise and recovery energy costs. A straight line also represents the geometry of choice for what's called a linear regression equation. Our previous statistical analyses of lifting to failure as compared to non-failure lifts utilized linear regression (straight line) comparisons between energy costs and work. One can also analyze things from non-linear perspectives.

Take a look at the next figure. In this example, the association between energy cost and work is <u>not</u> under-going examination. Instead, a ratio of work-to-cost is presented. Dismissing the default descriptor of a straight line, the statistical analysis program was told to draw *a line of best fit* through our work-to-cost representation of efficiency (the data provided are from the previous table; 1-set of lifts to muscular failure at a controlled lifting cadence of 3 seconds per repetition). The best fit line is a curved one, efficiency achieves a maximum with a greater number of repetitions as resistance training work increases:

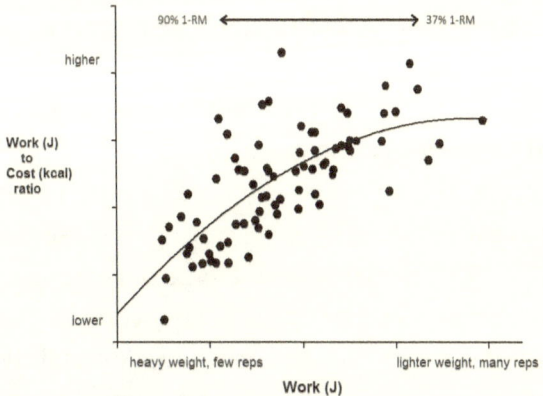

As more resistance exercise work is completed – muscular endurance, a lighter weight lifted more times - the work to energy cost ratio becomes more efficient, even as energy costs grow proportionately larger. This is true for both muscular failure and non-failure weight lifting conditions. Work is most inefficient when lifting a heavy weight with few repetitions. In fact, the curve mimics the oxygen uptake characteristics of a single bout of steady state aerobic exercise (not including recovery).

There are actually two interpretations at play here: 1) Energy costs increase as more resistance exercise work is completed and, 2) The work-to-cost relationship improves as more work is performed. What's going on here?

Dr. Herman Pontzer is an anthropologist who studies daily energy expenditure and his laboratory is currently the great outdoors. His findings are certainly not what anyone who wants to lose weight wants to hear: physically active people burn about the same number of calories per day as inactive people.

One rationalization for the observation of an increase in exercise energy costs for those who are physically active, while having daily energy costs that are similar for both active and sedentary folks, suggests that when physically active people are not moving about, resting energy needs are actually ratcheted down to minimize overall daily costs. I actually see elements of this interpretation within our own muscular endurance resistance exercise data where efficiency improves as repetitions increase.

Dr. Pontzer followed the daily energy costs of a true hunter-gatherer society that quite literally eats only what it can kill or harvest. These people may travel a dozen or so miles a day to track game; the tasks of harvesting likewise raise energy demands (I would consider them a type of endurance athlete). And yet the overall 24-hour daily energy costs of these people are about the same as you and me – that's certainly striking evidence to question the aptitude of an exercise program for the pursuit of weight loss.

As dictated by estimates of efficiency, our numbers reveal that total energy costs rise proportionately with increases in work or load as they should, but recovery (EPOC, afterburn) costs do not appear to follow suit. Recovery needs are indeed relatively high after brief high-load work bouts; this is the very protocol of choice for energy cost and fat burning maximization. However, moving from brief high-load work bouts to multiple repetition muscular endurance bouts that entail much more overall work (over a longer exercise time), the absolute recovery costs remain about the same for both – recovery costs actually begin to plateau as the amount of work increases.

So, should you be following an exercise routine where energy costs rise proportionately (linearly) with intensity or load? Or should you be focusing on inefficiency, where the cost-per-work ratio is maximized? My answers are yes. In terms of an exercise program that best maximizes caloric cost and fat burning I would choose simply:

Multiple brief intermittent bouts of heavy work (exercise) coupled with longer duration bouts of walking (recovery).

XIII.

Working Hypotheses

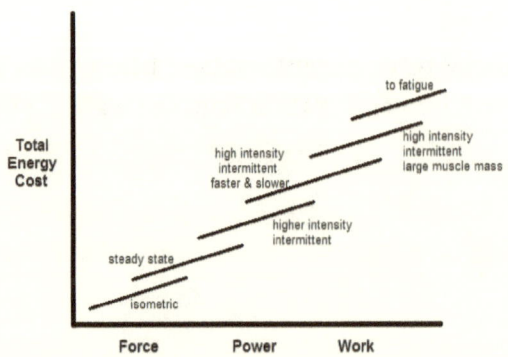

Linear depictions of energy costs are shown for isometric, steady state and intermittent work and recovery (these are not efficiency estimations). From isometric non-movement forces to steady state power output, to the conditions of intermittent exercise, a proportionately greater total energy cost is revealed, both within and among conditions as described within this text. Inefficiency is exploited with multiple, brief, high-load, bouts of intermittent exercise followed by extended recovery periods. If conditions change in terms of slower and faster movement speeds, a larger recruitment of working muscle mass and/or exercise to momentary muscular failure, total energy costs and fat burning will reach a maximum.

I am not a personal trainer, but the foundation of the energy cost and fat loss maximization game plans are provided below for those who are. Go and create! Here's a limited start...

Walking

Most able-bodied folks can perform this simple task, but how to maximize caloric costs and fat loss?

Improvements...

Intensity: Lifting one's body weight vertically adds to the overall work and energy cost. If you walk on a track that has bleachers, incorporate brief periods of stair-climbing. Better yet walk in a hilly area and power-up hills with exaggerated movements (remember, any change from your natural gait – rate, stride length, arm movement – will increase costs).

Intermittent exercise and larger muscle masses: Add a few to several whole-body calisthenics exercises after every several minutes of walking.

Track & Field

The quintessential example of aerobic
training; a 400 meter track.

Steady state: There is nothing wrong with steady state continuous walking or running, but caloric costs and fat burning can be better maximized.

Improvements:

Intermittent format: Brief sprinting periods attached to prolonged periods of walking or jogging may work best at burning fat-related calories.

Larger muscle group exercises: Incorporate brief periods of different forward-moving exercises into your walking or jogging routine, for example: hopping, skipping, leaping and more. Incorporate brief intense periods of large muscle group calisthenics (for example, burpees), followed by an extended walking/jogging recovery. Incorporate external loads into your routine, with equipment such as kettlebells, heavy ropes or good old-fashioned dumbbells and barbells.

Strongman-type Sports

Certainly not for beginners but even so, events like the Strongman truck/bus/car push/pull, best demonstrate those concepts required to maximize caloric costs:

Heavy weight: A weighted sled maybe more realistic than a truck/bus (push/pull).

Large muscle mass: The driving (pushing) of the legs in addition to the arms (pulling on a rope).

Speed: This is a competition, the fastest time wins. But play 'Bionic Man': try pushing and pulling that weight in slow motion.

Fatigue: A *competitor* should be at or close to failure at the end of the event.

Intermittent: As a strongman event the track consists of a 100-foot continuous push/pull. However, if broken down into several shorter intermittent exercise periods with each coupled to a few minutes of active walking recovery, fat burning and costs would be maximized.

Tire flip

Another example of a Strongman-type
activity, flipping a large heavy tire.

Intermittent: Brief periods of lifts or repetitions are preferred
with each coupled to minute(s) of an active walking recovery.
Complete multiple sets.

Heavy weight: The weight of the tire should be based on both
experience and fitness level.

Large muscle mass: Proper instruction/technique are requisite:
the all-important drive (pushing) of the legs in addition to the
arms (lifting upwards, then pushing forwards).

Speed: Either faster or slower as compared to a controlled
cadence.

XIV.

Not the End...

Our data currently portray *snapshots* of energy costs for a given type of physical task and we certainly have not and cannot test them all. Regardless, let's be honest with what's been found so far. While exercise certainly increases energy demands, its assistance in this department appears to be somewhat minimal to moderate from the vantage point of a single workout. Burning several hundred calories per workout is more in the realm of a professional athlete or fitness instructor who trains for a living. Regular physical movement certainly helps, but nutrition and diet need to be the primary focus of a weight loss program. Moreover, the possible negative impact of regular exercise for us ordinary folks - the potential *lowering* of caloric costs when you are not exercising, needs better understanding and application (perhaps fat burning is the more primary of adaptations).

Putting costs into perspective, let's say you set a reasonable goal of losing 1 pound of fat every 10 days. At 4,000 kcals per pound of fat that's a caloric expenditure of 400 kcal of exercise every day for 10 straight days. A rehashing of some of the exercises and tasks provided earlier is shown below and how each meets a **400 kcal of activity per day** protocol:

400 kcal based on **steady state per minute** methodology (recovery not included):

- Walking: 4 miles
- Cycling: ~60 minutes at 6 mph
  ~30 minutes at 15 mph

400 kcal based on **cost per task** methodology (exercise and recovery):

- Isometric squat Tabata routine: 26 four-minute routines (with a minutes long recovery period after each routine)
- Heavy bag punching: 13 all-out one-minute rounds (with 13 recovery periods)
- 250 watts cycling: 14 one-minute sprints (with 14 recovery periods)
- Calisthenic All-out Tabata routine: 6 four-minute routines (burpee's and lunges with a minutes long recovery period after each routine)
- Resistance exercise muscular endurance: 26 sets of bench press, 30+ reps per set - each to muscular failure (37% 1-RM, ~900 overall repetitions, 47 minutes of exercise) (plus 26 recovery periods)
- Resistance exercise strength training: 50 sets of bench press, 4 reps per set - each to muscular failure (90% 1-RM, 200 overall repetitions, 20 minutes of exercise with 100 recovery periods)
- Resistance exercise lifting to failure: 18 sets of squats (50% 1-RM, ~360 overall repetitions).

In brief, 1) the caloric costs of many intense exercise programs are probably not as high as you would like them to be, 2) regular exercise does not appear to increase daily energy demands all that much and 3) performing most of the above tasks would almost certainly result in injury.

Some may find these conclusions depressing and ask, "why even bother to exercise in the first place?" Here's why. I've been involved with the health and well-being 'industry' for some time now and have discussed with many a colleague and client the consequences of poor behavior. That is, behavior we actually choose to engage in. And perhaps the single worst behavior is choosing to be sedentary: I know that, Dr. Pontzer knows that, Jack LaLanne and Richard Simmons knew that…it needs to be incorporated into the psyche of everyone.

While caloric expenditure may not be at a premium, physical movement is nothing short of a miracle worker when it comes to health and physiological development: Fitness! Physical performance! Strength, speed, power! But this is not a book about that. The image of well-muscled, red-faced, instructors pleading into the ears of overweight clients - "KEEP GOING, ONE MORE!" – needs to change.

No doubt, due to the diligent work of exercise scientists and personal trainers, all of whom I would call colleagues, a valid knowledge of the weight loss characteristics for every and all kinds of activity, especially higher intensity intermittent exercise, will indeed improve over time. At the moment I am unsure as to what ratio of exercise-to-recovery times would work best for actual weight loss, but I am hopeful that brief bouts of whole-body, higher intensity/load, intermittent exercise designed from a format of inefficiency (increased costs) coupled to longer duration, lower intensity, aerobic steady state, active recovery periods (increased fat burning) is the best approach.

Of course, individual responses – both physiological and psychological - may likely vary to an extent that program design will need to differ for all involved, each format being individually tailored to best suit that particular individual. Whatever your level of understanding is with exercise program design, I'm under the impression that the following synopsis would be accepted by almost all: exercise enthusiast, fitness specialist, scientist or dietician:

In an attempt to maximize energy costs and fat burning, there are a myriad of advantages to brief higher intensity or load intermittent training as compared to steady state exercise formats.

Bibliography

Introduction

ACSM's Guidelines for Exercise Testing and Prescription, 9th Ed. Lippincott, Williams & Wilkins: Baltimore, MD., 2014.

Kokkinos, P. Physical activity, health benefits, and mortality risk. *ISRN Cardiology.* Doi:10.5402/2012/18789, 2012.

Laursen, P.B. and Jenkins, D.G. The scientific basis for high-intensity interval training: optimizing training programs and maximizing performance in highly trained endurance athletes. *Sports Medicine.* 32:53-73, 2002.

Pontzer, H. The Exercise Paradox. *Scientific American.* 316:26-31, 2017.

Roberts, S.B. and Das, S.K. The messy truth about weight loss. *Scientific American.* 316:36-41, 2017.

Move!

Borg, G. Perceived exertion as an indicator of somatic stress. *Scandinavian Journal of Rehabilitation and Medicine.* 2: 92–8, 1970.

DeLooze, M.P., Toussaint, H.M., Commissaris, D.A., Jans, M.P. and Sargeant, A.J. Relationships between energy expenditure and positive and negative mechanical work in repetitive lifting and lowering. *Journal of Applied Physiology.* 77:420-426, 1994.

McArdle, W.D. and Foglia, G.F. Energy cost and cardiorespiratory stress of isometric and weight training exercises. *Journal of Sports Medicine and Physical Fitness.* 9:23-30, 1969.

Roberts, T.J. Contribution of elastic tissues to the mechanics and energetics of muscle function during movement. *Journal of Experimental Biology.* 219: 266-275, 2016.

Scott, C.B., Nelson, E., Martin, S. and Ligotti, B. Total energy costs of 3 Tabata-type calisthenic squatting routines: isometric, isotonic and jump, *European Journal of Human Movement*, 35: 34-40, 2015.

Law of the Land: The Aerobic Steady State Energy Cost

ACSM's Guidelines for Exercise Testing and Prescription, 9th Ed. Lippincott, Williams & Wilkins: Baltimore, MD., 2014.

Cooper, K.H. *Aerobics.* M. Evans and Co. publ. (Lippincott, Phil.), 1968.

Passmore, R. and Durnin J.V.G.A. Human energy expenditure. *Physiological Reviews.* 35:801-840, 1955.

Steudel-Numbers, K.L. and Wall-Scheffler, C.M. Optimal running speed and the evolution of hominin hunting strategies. *Journal of Human Evolution.* 65:355-360, 2009.

Taylor, R.C. Relating mechanics and energetics during exercise. *Advances in Veterinary Science and Comparative Medicine.* 38A:181-215, 1994.

No-Man's Land: The Anaerobic Threshold

Antonutto, G. and Di Prampero, P.E. The concept of the anaerobic threshold: a short review. *Journal of Sports Medicine and Physical Fitness.* 35:6-12, 1995.

Brooks, G.A. Anaerobic threshold: review of the concept and directions for future research. *Medicine and Science in Sports and Exercise.* 17:22-31, 1985.

Faude, O., Kindermann, W. and Meyer, T. Lactate threshold concepts: how valid are they? *Sports Medicine.* 39:469-490, 2009.

Keith, S.P., Jacobs, I. and McLellan, T.M. Adaptations to training at the individual anaerobic threshold. *European Journal of Applied Physiology.* 65:316-323, 1992.

A Different Perspective: Energy Cost per Task

Mazzetti, S., M. Douglass, A. Yocum and Harber, M. Effect of explosive versus slow contractions and exercise intensity on energy expenditure. *Medicine and Science in Sports Exercise.* 39:1291-1301, 2007.

Scott, C.B. The effect of time-under-tension and weight lifting cadence on aerobic, anaerobic, and recovery energy expenditures: 3 submaximal sets. *Applied Physiology Nutrition and Metabolism.* 37:252-256, 2012.

Scott, C.B., N.D. Littlefield, J.D. Chason, M.P. Bunker and E.M. Asselin. Aerobic and anaerobic energy expenditure for brief equivalent bouts of cycling and running. *Nutrition and Metabolism.* 3:1, 2006.

Steudel-Numbers, K.L. and Wall-Scheffler, C.M. Optimal running speed and the evolution of hominin hunting strategies. *Journal of Human Evolution.* 65:355-360, 2009.

Stop and Go: Intermittent Exercise

Adams, E., Allen, N.B., Schumm, J.E. and Swank, A.M. Oxygen cost of boxing exercise utilizing a heavy bag. *Medicine and Science in Sport and Exercise.* 29: S187, 1993.

Ainsworth B.E., Haskell, W.L., Whitt, M.C., Irwin, M.L., Swartz, A.N., Strath, S.J., O'Brien, W.L., Bassett, D.R., Schmitz, K.H., Emplaincourt, P.O., Jacobs, D.R. and Leon, A.S. Compendium of physical activities: an update of activity codes and MET intensities. *Medicine and Science in Sport and* Exercise. 32: S498-S516, 2000.

Arseneau, E., Mekary, S. and Leger, L. VO2 requirements of boxing exercises. *J Strength Cond Res.* 2011; 25: 348-359

Bahr, R. Excess post-exercise oxygen consumption – magnitude, mechanisms and practical implications. *Acta Physiologica Scandinavia.* 144: Supplement 605, 1992.

Borsheim, E. and Bahr, R. Effect of exercise intensity, duration and mode on post-exercise oxygen consumption. *Sports Medicine.* 33:1037-1060, 2003.

Boutcher, S.H. High-intensity intermittent exercise and fat loss. *Journal of Obesity.* article ID 868305, 2011.

Burleson, M.A., O'Bryant, H.S., Stone, M.H., Collins, M.A. and Triplett-McBride, T. Effect of weight training exercise and treadmill exercise on elevated post-exercise oxygen consumption. *Medicine and Science in Sports and Exercise.* 30:518-522, 1998.

Essen, B. Studies on the regulation of metabolism in human skeletal muscle using intermittent exercise as an experimental model. *Acta Physiologica Scandinavia.* Supplement.454:1-32, 1978.

Gaesser, G.A. and Brooks, G.A. Metabolic basis of excess post-exercise oxygen consumption; a review. *Medicine and Science in Sports and Exercise.* 16:29-43, 1984.

Henderson, G.C., Fattor, J.A., Horning, M.A., Faghihnia, N., Johnson, M.L., Mau, T.L., Luke-Zeitoun, M. and Brooks, G.A. Lipolysis and fatty acid metabolism in men and women during the postexercise recovery period. *Journal of Physiology.* 584.3:963-981, 2007.

Kuo, C.C., Fattor, J.A., Henderson, G.C. and Brooks, G.A. Lipid oxidation in fit young adults during postexercise recovery. *Journal of Applied Physiology.* 99:349-356, 2005.

O'Driscoll, E., Steele, J., Perez, H., Yreys, S., Snowkroft, N. and Locasio, F. The metabolic cost of two trials of boxing exercise utilizing a heavy bag. *Medicine and Science in Sports and Exercise.* 31: S158, 1999.

Scott, C.B. Combustion, respiration and intermittent exercise: a theoretical perspective on oxygen uptake and energy expenditure. *Biology.* 3:255-263, 2014.

Scott, C.B. Glucose and fat oxidation: bomb calorimeter be damned. *Scientific World Journal.* Article ID 375041, 2012.

Mulla, N.A.L., Simonsen, L. and Bulow, J. Post-exercise adipose tissue and skeletal muscle lipid metabolism in humans: the effects of exercise intensity. *Journal of Physiology.* 524.3:919-928, 2000.

HIIT Me: Higher Intensity Intermittent Training (aerobic)

Balsom, P.D, Seger, J.Y., Sjodin, B. and Ekblom, B. Physiological responses to maximal intensity intermittent exercise. *European Journal of Applied Physiology.* 65: 144-149, 1992.

Boutcher, S.H. High-intensity intermittent exercise and fat loss. *Journal of Obesity.* 2011. Doi:10.1155/2011/868305

Christensen, E.H., Hedman, R. and Saltin, B. Intermittent and continuous running. *Acta Physiologica Scandinavia.* 50:269-286, 1960.

De Feo, P. Is high-intensity exercise better than moderate-intensity exercise for weight loss? *Nutrition, Metabolism and Cardiovascular Diseases.* 23:1037-1042, 2013.

Edwards, R.H.T., D.K. Hill and McDonnell, M. Myothermal and intramuscular pressure measurements during isometric contractions of the human quadriceps muscle. *Journal of Physiology*. 224:58P-59P, 1972.

Foster, C., Farland, C.V., Guidotti, F., Harbin, M., Roberts, B., Schuette, J., Tuuri, A., Doberstein, S.T., and Porcari, J.P. The effects of high intensity interval training vs steady state training on aerobic and anaerobic capacity. *Journal of Sports Science and Medicine*. 14: 747-755, 2015.

Gaitanos, G.C., Williams, C., Boobis, L.H. and Brooks, S. Human muscle metabolism during intermittent maximal exercise. *Journal of Applied Physiology*. 75: 712-719, 1993.

Gibala, M.J. and McGee, S.L. Metabolic adaptations to short-term high-intensity interval training: a little pain for a lot of gain? Exercise and Sport Science Reviews. 36:58-63, 2008.

Islam, H., Townsend, L.K., and Hazell, T.J. Modified sprint training interval protocols. Part I. Physiological responses. *Applied Physiology, Nutrition and Metabolism*. 42:339-346, 2017.

Hunter, G. R., R.I. Weinsier, M.M. Bamman and Larson, D.E. A role for high intensity exercise on energy balance and weight control. *International Journal of Obesity*. 22:489-493, 1998.

Laursen, P.B. and Jenkins, D.G. The scientific basis for high-intensity interval training. *Sports Medicine*. 32: 53-73, 2002.

Tabata, I., Nishimira, M., Kouzaki, M. et al. Effects of moderate intensity-endurance and high intensity-intermittent training on anaerobic capacity and VO_{2max}. *Medicine and Science in Sports and Exercise*. 28: 1327-1330, 1996.

Tabata, I., Irisawa, K., Kouzaki, M., Nishimura, K., Ogita, F. and Miyachi, M. Metabolic profile of high intensity intermittent exercises. *Medicine and Science in Sports and Exercise.* 29:390-395, 1997.

Townsend, L.K., Islam, H., Dunn, E., Eys, M., Robertson-Wilson, J. and Hazell, T.J. Modified sprint training interval protocols. Part II. Psychological responses. *Applied Physiology, Nutrition and Metabolism.* 42:347-353, 2017.

Strongman: Heavy Load Intermittent Exercise (anaerobic)

Binzen, C.A., Swan, P.D. and Manore, M.M. Postexercise oxygen consumption and substrate use after resistance exercise in women. *Medicine and Science in Sports and Exercise.* 33:932-938, 2001.

Burd, N.A., West, D.W.D., Staples, A.W., Atherton, P.J., Baker, J.M., Moore, D.R., Holwerda, A.M., Parise, G., Rennie, M.J., Baker, S.K. and Phillips, S.M. Low-load high volume resistance exercise stimulates muscle protein synthesis more than high-load low volume resistance exercise in young men. PLOS ONE. August 9, 2010.

Cook, C.J., Kilduff, L.P. and Beaven, C.M. Improving strength and power in trained athletes with 3 weeks of occlusion training. *International Journal of Sports Physiology and Performance.* 9:166-172, 2014.

Edwards, R.H.T., Hill, D.K. and McDonnell, M. Myothermal and intramuscular pressure measurements during isometric contractions of the human quadriceps muscle. *Journal of Physiology.* 224:58P-59P, 1972.

Farinatti, P., A.G.C. Neto and N.L. da Silva. Influence of resistance training variables on excess postexercise oxygen consumption: a systematic review. *ISRN Physiology.* Article ID: 825026. 2013.

Manini, T.M. and Clark, B.C. Blood flow restricted exercise and skeletal muscle health. *Exercise and Sport Science Reviews.* 37:78-85, 2009.

McArdle, W.D. and Foglia, G.F. Energy cost and cardiorespiratory stress of isometric and weight training exercises. *Journal of Sports Medicine and Physical Fitness.* 9:23-30, 1969.

Meirelles, C. dM. and Gomes, P.S.C. Acute effects of resistance exercise on energy expenditure: revisiting the impact of the training variables. *Revista Brasileira do Medicina do Esporte.* 10:131-138, 2004.

Melby, C., C. Scholl, G. Edwards and R. Bullough. Effects of acute resistance exercise on post-exercise energy expenditure and resting metabolic rate. *Journal of Applied Physiology.* 75:1847-1853, 1993.

Ormsbee, M.J., Thyfault, J.P., Johnson, E.A., Kraus, R.M., Choi, M.D. and Hickner, R.C. Fat metabolism and acute exercise in trained men. *Journal of Applied Physiology.* 102:1767-1772, 2007.

Scott, C.B. Quantifying the immediate recovery energy expenditure of resistance exercise. *Journal of Strength and Conditioning Research.* 25:1159-1163, 2011.

Scott, C.B., Leary, M.P. and TenBraak, A.J. Energy expenditure characteristics of weight lifting: 2 sets to fatigue. *Applied Physiology Nutrition and Metabolism*. 36:115-120, 2011.

Scott, C.B. Oxygen costs peak after resistance exercise sets: a rationale for the importance of recovery over exercise. *Journal of Exercise Physiology online*. 15:1-8, 2012.

Scott, C.B. The effect of time-under-tension and weight lifting cadence on aerobic, anaerobic, and recovery energy expenditures: 3 submaximal sets. *Applied Physiology Nutrition and Metabolism*. 37:252-256, 2012.

Steele, J., Fisher, J., McGuff, D., Bruce-Low, S. and Smith, D. Resistance training to momentary muscular failure improves cardiovascular fitness in humans. A review of acute physiological responses and chronic physiological adaptations. *Journal of Exercise Physiology online*. 15:53-80, 2012.

Tamaki, T., Uchiyama, S., Tamura, T. and Nakano, S. Changes in muscle oxygenation during weight-lifting exercise. *European Journal of Applied Physiology*. 68:465-469, 1994.

Vilaca-Alves, J., Freitas, N.M., Saavedra, F.J., Scott, C.B., Reis, V.M., Simao, R. and Garrido, N. Comparison of oxygen uptake during and after the execution of resistance exercises and exercises performed on ergometers, matched for intensity. *Journal of Human Kinetics*. 53:179-187, 2016.

Think Big: Large Muscle Groups

Scott, C.B., A. Luchini, A. Knausenberger and Steitz, A. Total energy costs – aerobic and anaerobic, exercise and recovery – of five resistance exercises. *Central European Journal of Sport Sciences and Medicine.* 8: 53-59, 2014.

Paying for Pain: Muscle Failure

Jung, M.E., Bourne, J.E. and Little, J.P. Where does HIT fit? An examination of the affective response to high-intensity intervals in comparison to continuous moderate- and vigorous-intensity exercise in the exercise intensity-continuum. *PLoS ONE.* 2014. DOI: 10.1371/journal.pone.0114541.

Parfitt, G. and Hughes, S. The exercise intensity-affect relationship: evidence and implications for exercise behavior. *Journal of Exercise Science and Fitness.* 7:S34-S41, 2009.

Scott, C.B. and Earnest, C.P. Resistance exercise energy expenditure is greater with fatigue as compared to non-fatigue. *Journal of Exercise Physiology online.* 14:1-10, 2011.

Do it for Health

ACSM's Guidelines for Exercise Testing and Prescription, 9th Ed. Lippincott, Williams & Wilkins: Baltimore, MD., 2014.

Gillen, J.B., Martin, B.J., Macinnis, M.J., Skelly, L.E., Taropolsky, M.A. and Gibala, M.J. Twelve weeks of sprint interval training improves indices of cardiometabolic health similar to traditional endurance training despite a five-fold lower exercise volume and time commitment. PLoS ONE 11(4): e0154075. DOI:10.1371/journal.pone.0154075.

Kokkinos, P. Physical activity, health benefits, and mortality risk. *ISRN Cardiology.* Doi:10.5402/2012/18789, 2012.

Seidell, J.C., Muller, D.C., Sorkin, J.D. and Andres, R. Fasting respiratory exchange ratio and resting metabolic rate as predictors of weight gain: the Baltimore longitudinal study on aging. *International Journal of Obesity.* 16: 667-674, 1992.

Graber, C. and Twilley, N. Why the calorie is broken. *Mosiacscience.com* January 26, 2016.

Harcombe, Z. Designed by the food industry for wealth not health: the "Eatwell Guide". *British Journal of Sports Medicine.* doi:10.1136/bjsports-2016-096297.

Adamson, S., Lorimer, R., Cobley, J.M., Lloyd, R. and Babraj, J. High intensity training improves health and physical function in middle aged adults. *Biology.* 3: 333-334, 2014.

Chowdhury, R., Warnakula, S., Kunutsor, S., Crowe, F., Ward, H.A., Johnson, L., Franco, O.H., Butterworth, A.S., Forouhi, N.G., Thompson, S.G., Khaw, K-T., Mozaffarian, D., Danesh, J. and Di Angelantonio, D. Association of dietary, circulating and supplement fatty acids with coronary risk: a systematic review and meta-analysis. *Annals of Internal Medicine.* 160:398-406, 2014.

Earnest, C.P. Exercise interval training: an improved stimulus for improving the physiology of pre-diabetes. *Medical Hypotheses.* 71:752-761, 2008.

Earnest, C.P., Johannsen, N.M., Swift, D.L., Gillison, F.B., Mikus, C.R., Lucia, A., Kramer, K., Lavie, C.J. and Church, T.S. Aerobic and strength training in concomitant metabolic syndrome and type 2 diabetes. *Medicine and Science in Sport and Exercise.* 46:1293-1301, 2014.

Fix, J.F. *The Complete Book of Running.* Random House Publ. 1977.

Heydari, M., Freund, J. and Boutcher, S.H. The effect of high-intensity intermittent exercise on body composition of overweight young males. *Journal of Obesity*. Article ID 480467. 2012.

Paoli, A., Moro, T., Marcolin, G., Neri, M., Bianco, A., Palma, A. and Grimaldi, K. High-intensity interval resistance training (HIRT) influences resting energy expenditure and respiratory ratio in non-dieting individuals. *Journal of Translational Medicine*. 10:237,, 2012.

Paoli, A., Oacelli, Q.F., Moro, T., Marcolin, G., Neri,, M., Battaglia, G., Sergi, G., Bolzetta, F. and Bianco, A. Effects of high-intensity circuit training, low-intensity circuit training and endurance training on blood pressure and lipoproteins in middle-aged overweight men. *Lipids in Health and Disease*. 12:131, 2013.

Roberts, B.H. http://www.thedailybeast.com/articles/2014/05/22/the-heart-association-s-junk-science-diet.html

An Exercise Science Lab

Pontzer, H. The Exercise Paradox. *Scientific American*. 316:26-31, 2017.

Scott, C.B., Leighton, B.H., Ahearn, K.J. and McManus, J.J. Aerobic, anaerobic and excess post-exercise oxygen consumption energy expenditure of muscular endurance and strength: 1-set of bench press to muscular fatigue. *Journal of Strength and Conditioning Research*. 25:903-908, 2011.

Scott, C.B. and Earnest, C.P. Resistance exercise energy expenditure is greater with fatigue as compared to non-fatigue. *Journal of Exercise Physiology online.* 14:1-10, 2011.

Scott, C.B., Leary, M.P. and TenBraak, A.J. Energy expenditure characteristics of weight lifting: 2 sets to fatigue. *Applied Physiology Nutrition and Metabolism.* 36:115-120, 2011.

Scott, C.B. and Reis, V. Steady state models provide an invalid estimate of intermittent resistance-exercise energy costs. *European Journal of Human Movement.* 33:70-78, 2014.

Scott, C.B. and Reis, V.M. Modeling the total energy costs of resistance exercise: a work in progress. *Central European Journal of Sports Science and Medicine* 14:5-12, 2016.

Not the End...

Islam, H., Townsend, L.K., and Hazell, T.J. Modified sprint training interval protocols. Part I. Physiological responses. *Applied Physiology, Nutrition and Metabolism.* 42:339-346, 2017.

Melby, C. and Hickey, M. Energy balance and body weight regulation. *Sports Science Exchange* (Gatorade Sports Science Institute), 18:1-6, 2005.

Scott, C.B. The biology of exercise and weight loss: Fat oxidation compels oxygen uptake. *Biology* 2018 (in press).

Townsend, L.K., Islam, H., Dunn, E., Eys, M., Robertson-Wilson, J. and Hazell, T.J. Modified sprint training interval protocols. Part II. Psychological responses. *Applied Physiology, Nutrition and Metabolism.* 42:347-353, 2017.

Acknowledgements

None of the material presented here would have come into existence without the commitment and dedication of those Exercise Physiology majors within the University of Southern Maines' Exercise, Health and Sports Science program – an undergraduate student program. While Senior year students can choose to complete a thesis project of their own design, many adhered to the energy cost theme that our Human Performance Lab has often focused. They were the crux of a data collecting collaboration that I cannot be more proud of.

The first draft of this manuscript was initially about 200 pages in length, nearly twice that of the final outcome. As with this text, it was intended for all audiences. A few former undergraduate classmates, including Dana Murgita, read it and appeared somewhat pleased but not overly excited with my accomplishment. But Will Watman and Dennis Morton, both family friends long retired, gave me blunter news. Based on their feedback, I removed almost 100 pages of material and rewrote the entirety of what was left. Will also reviewed the latter manuscript along with Kevin Gallagher and Craig Grover. My greatest appreciation goes to who I would consider my official editor Tracey Mousseau, her expertise and commitment were welcomed.

The loving support of my wife – Martha Scott – must also be mentioned. Martha continues to be immensely supportive of University and student-related research, especially with the often outrageous time commitments (and sometimes financial assistance) required of the many projects that I have mentored.

About the Author

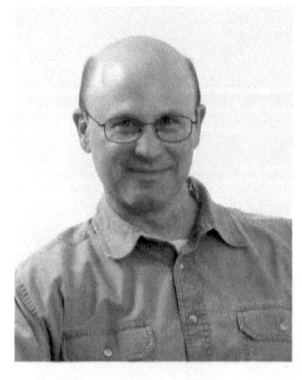

Christopher B. Scott, PhD, is an exercise physiologist with a thirty-five year career in fitness, science, medicine, and academia. His current teaching priorities reside within the Exercise Science program at the University of Southern Maine with a research agenda that focuses on the estimation of the energy costs of strength, speed, and power-related exercise and activities. He has published more than sixty research-related articles in peer-reviewed journals, and his findings on how exercise best contributes to weight loss have been presented worldwide.

www.ingramcontent.com/pod-product-compliance
Lightning Source LLC
Chambersburg PA
CBHW020540290526
45786CB00002B/977